All truth passes through three stages:

First, it is ridiculed.

Second, it is violently opposed.

Third, it is accepted as self-evident.

--Source Unknown

FDA REQUIRED DISCLAIMER:

This book is for educational purposes and is not intended to be used as a substitute for the diagnosis, treatment and advice of a qualified licensed medical professional.

This book offers people medical information and tells them their alternative medical options, but in no way should anyone consider that the author or this book represents the "practice of medicine."

The author assumes no responsibility for how the information in this book is used.

Further, alternative treatments for disease and cancer are constantly being discovered and some of the alternative treatments in this book may not be available or have become outdated or banned.

Finally, my statements and those of others regarding alternative treatments for disease and cancer have not been evaluated by the FDA.

ALTERNATIVE REVELATIONS

3rd Edition

"The Source for Medical Freedom"

by

LJ Emmanuel

Copyright 2016 The Wintermantel Group LLC
All rights reserved

Published by CreateSpace (Amazon.com)
www.createspace.com
First Edition ISBN 978-1480074095
Second Edition ISBN 978-1505257540
Third Edition ISBN 978-1541069145
December 11, 2016

No part of this publication/book may be duplicated or copied in any format without the written permission of the author.

I cannot be responsible for broken or scrubbed website links.

For more information visit www.lindaemmanuel.com

SECTION 1 – "REDEFINING"

Cancer and Disease Facts and Stats (2016) 11
A Worldwide Epidemic of Cancer and Disease 12
An Explanation as to "Why" 13
US Patent on Mycoplasma 16
"The Third Time's a Charm" 18
The Driving Forces behind the Epidemic 19
Mycoplasma Q&A 21
Symptoms of a Mycoplasma Infection 26
Mycoplasma Literature 28
More Facts about Mycoplasma 36
Anemia and Mycoplasma 39
Nitric Oxide 43
Mycoplasma, Nitric Oxide and ADMA 45
The Truth about Heart Disease 47
Mycoplasma and the Cachexia Cycle 50
Mycoplasma, Nagalase and GcMAF 52
Mycoplasma and Vaccines 55
Lyme Disease 57

SECTION 2 – "BALANCING"

Introduction 63
It's No Acid-ent Why Some People Do Not Get Sick 65
Vegetable pH Table 67
Fruit pH Table 68
Miscellaneous pH Table 69
The Gerson Therapy 70
Fat, Sick and Nearly Dead 72
Baking Soda 73
The Story of Vernon "Vito" Johnson 74
The Story of Dr. Simoncini 76

Baking Soda and Lemon Juice Protocol 77
Six Lemons a Day Keep the Mycoplasma Away Protocol 78
Baking Soda and Maple Syrup Protocol... 79
Calcium Protocol 80

SECTION 3 – "DETOXING"

Sulfur 82
Tony Isaac's Liver Cleanse Protocol 83
Ion Footbath 84
The Story of Dr. Hazel Parcells.. 85
The Parcells Oxygen Soak... 86

SECTION 4 – "PROTECTING"

The Ketogenic Diet.. 88
Bovine Colostrum 90
The Story of AZOMITE... 93
Diatomaceous Earth 95

SECTION 5 – "DEFENDING"

Introduction 100
1. Alkaloids 101
2. Glucosinolates... 104
3. Cyanogenic Glycosides 106
    Sources of Cyanogenic Glycosides 107
    Amygdalin... 108
    Flaxseed.. 110
    Flaxseed Protocol 111
    Flaxseed Oil and Oil of Oregano Protocol.................................... 112
4. Sulfur 113
    Onions... 114
    Garlic 115
    Asparagus.. 117
    Asparagus Protocol 119

5. Medium-Chain Fatty Acids 120

SECTION 6 – "KILLING"

Tobacco 128
Marijuana (Hemp) 129
The Truth about Marijuana 133
The Story of Hemp-Eze 136
Hemp Seeds 138
Cat's Claw 141
Oleander 142
Vinca Minor 144
Vinca Minor Protocol 145
Goldenseal 147
Marigold 148
Essiac Tea 149
Hoxsey Therapy 152
Bloodroot 155
The Truth about Cinnamon 157
Cinnamon Protocol 159
Turmeric 160
Ginger 161
Ginger/Turmeric Protocol 162
Castor Oil 163
Castor Oil Protocol 167
Venus Flytrap 168
A Medicinal Garden 170
The Rife Machine 175
The Zapper 178
Silver (Ag) 179
Colloidal Silver 181
Mild Silver Protein 182

Sulfur 184
Vitamin C Therapy 186
Do-It-Yourself Vitamin C 190
John Beard, Father of Enzyme Therapy 191
The Truth about Enzyme Therapy 194
Forks Over Knives 196
PDQ Skin Cream 197
Heat Therapy 198
Aromatherapy 200
Phage Therapy 202
Summary 205
Sources 206
Definition of Wisdom 211

****

Section 1

"Redefining" Cancer and Disease

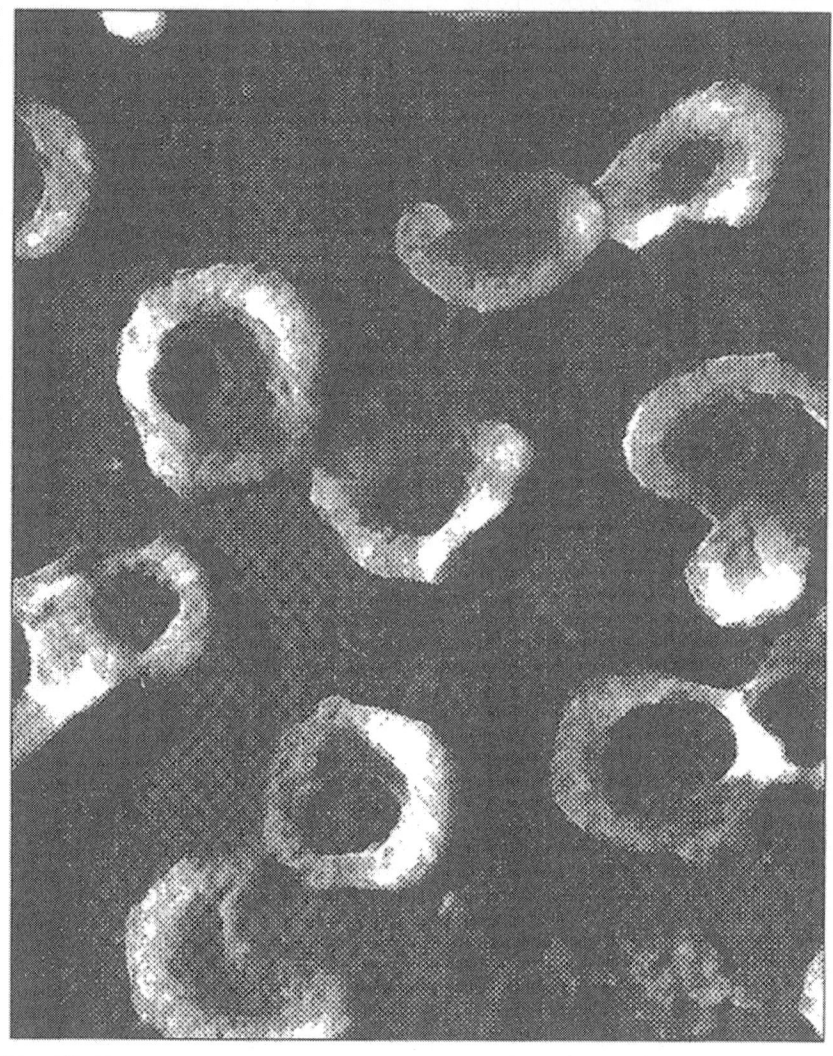

Mycoplasmas
80,000 x magnification

Cancer and Disease Facts and Stats (2016)

ALZHEIMER'S
- (US) In 2016 more than 5 million

FIBROMYALGIA
- Five million Americans have Fibromyalgia (95% women)

BREAST CANCER
- In 2016 300,000 new cases are expected

COLON/RECTAL CANCER
- In 2016, second leading cause of cancer deaths.

DIABETES
- (Source: CDC) 29.1 million Americans have diabetes

PROSTATE CANCER
- The most common cancer in men

MULTIPLE SCLEROSIS
- More than 400,000 Americans have MS

HEART DISEASE
- Leading cause of death in the US

LUNG CANCER
- #1 (1 in 4) cause of cancer deaths

BI-POLAR/CHRONIC DEPRESSION
- Affects 15+ million US adults; 250 million worldwide

PARKINSON'S
- (US) 60,000 new cases a year
- One million in US and 10 million worldwide

(The above statistics were gathered from cancer/disease foundations and government agency web sites. The above diseases and cancer are related to mycoplasma.)

A Worldwide Epidemic of Cancer and Disease

In the mid-1980s, Medicare set new policy. No longer would a patient be in the hospital for just tests. Ex: Gallbladder surgery—you were an outpatient or just stayed overnight. It was the same for any simple surgery. Major surgery, you were probably out within a couple of days with drainage tubes still in you to be taken care of by a visiting nurse.

Worse yet, insurance companies adopted Medicare's policy.

In the late 1980s, hospitals were in a dilemma. Beds were empty. Frantic, hospitals had to do what they had to do—they began downsizing—laying off employees and closing hospital wings.

It was around this time that nurses began working 12-hour shifts. People who were now in the hospital were very sick. Instead of taking care of a floor with just a few very sick people, nurses were overwhelmed with extremely sick patients needing serious care. Nurses were "burning out" and they were quitting, causing a nursing shortage.

Now, let's fast forward to 2016. Hospitals are booming, expanding and building more and more wings. The medical industry is where all the jobs are. Hospital parking lots are jammed. Doctors' waiting rooms are filled. It takes six weeks to see a specialist. There is an epidemic of autoimmune diseases. Heart disease is the #1 killer in America. Cancer is on the rise. Lyme disease has now reached epidemic proportions.

Cancer and disease are now "big" business in the US. According to Marcia Angell, the author of *The Truth About the Drug Companies:*

> "In 2002 the combined profits for the ten drug companies in the Fortune 500 were more than the profits for <u>all</u> the other 490 companies combined."

NOTE: And that was fourteen years ago! Can you imagine what it is today? What happened?

The next chapter explains "why" we are experiencing an epidemic of cancer and disease.

An Explanation as to "Why"

Officially the US bio-weapon program started in the 1930s with Rockefeller studies of population growth and how to limit it. The first pathogen (polio) to be tested was dispersed through aerosol in a Los Angeles hospital. Unfortunately, 200 of the 1500 hospital nurses and doctors were disabled from this polio "test." (Source: *The Brucellosis Triangle* by Donald W. Scott and William Scott.)

It was not until after World War II that the US government began earnestly concentrating on a more virulent bio-weapon, in particular the Brucellosis bacterium. This bacterium could jump species, i.e., from goats to humans or cows to humans. The Brucellosis bacteria could attack any and all body systems.

This was by far a nasty debilitating pathogen, but fortunately, bacteria are too large to cross the blood-brain barrier and can be detected by the immune system.

In the meantime, our government designated Fort Detrick, Maryland as the site to develop bio-weapons.

Their objective was a bio-weapon that would go "undetected" by the immune system and disable and/or kill its host. Of course, the perfect bio-weapon was mycoplasma, a cell-wall deficient bacterium—the smallest living organism. It is the genetic material of a bacterium encased in a membrane. However, the Brucellosis bacteria had a cell wall and could be detected by the immune system.

The following is a quote from Donald W. Scott's *The Brucellosis Triangle*, where he exposed the US government's bio-weapon program:

> "One of the pathogens which received extensive attention was brucellosis, and by 1946 the Fort Dietrick biological warfare researchers had developed the capability of producing thousands of gallons of the bacteria per month, and they had also developed the ability to produce the toxin* from the bacteria in a crystalline form. The agent was designed as a disabling agent and several tests were necessary to get it right, as Dr. MacArthur had acknowledged on June 9, 1969."

*Toxin = Mycoplasma or the nucleus of the Bucellosis bacterium

Once they learned how to extract and crystallize mycoplasma from the Bucellosis bacterium, the next step was to grind it up for disbursement whether it was through aerosol, vectors, chemtrails, or the food chain.

According to the Common Cause Medical Research Foundation, the following are documented mycoplasma bio-weapon "tests" on the general population:

- Iceland (1947-1948) – Over 1,000 victims, including five teenagers who all developed Parkinson's and later died.
- Punta Gorda, Florida (1956) Mosquitoes used as vectors. (The first cases of Chronic Fatigue Syndrome and Fibromyalgia were seen in America.)
- Korean War - It disabled 100's of thousands of North Koreans and Chinese troops, plus over 2,000 American troops.
- Tahoe-Truckee High School (1984) Mycoplasma fermentan incognito was released through aerosol in the high school vents. (Source: *Osler's Web* by Hillary Johnson)

According to Donald W. Scott, the founder of the Common Cause Medical Research Foundation, the head of the bio-weapon program at Fort Dietrick (Dr. MacArthur) told congress that this bio-weapon (mycoplasma) was not transmitted through secondary aerosol, but he was wrong. It could be spread through sharing and breathing the same air with an infected person (airplanes).

In fact, mycoplasmas can reside comfortably in the upper respiratory tract, the urinary tract and the intestinal tract. Mycoplasma infections are easily transmitted through sex (sharing body fluids).

The government filed for a patent on this "new" genetically modified Brucellosis bacterium, calling it Mycoplasma Fermentan Incognito.

U.S. PATENT

In the body of the US Patent filed on June 6, 1991 by the US Army for the pathogen mycoplasma fermentans incognitus, it states:

> "Some of these patients who are infected with M. Fermentans Incognitus will be patients who have been diagnosed as having AIDS or ARC, Chronic Fatigue Syndrome, Wegener's Disease, Sarcoidosis, respiratory distress syndrome, Kibuchi's disease, autoimmune diseases such as Collagen Vascular disease and Lupus and chronic debilitating diseases such as Alzheimer's disease."

On the next page is a (partial) photocopy of the US patent, which appeared in the Common Cause Medical Research Foundation's journal entitled, *AIDS: Made in America.*

Shyh-Ching Lo's Patent of the Pathogenic Mycoplasma

United States Patent [19]

Lo

[54] PATHOGENIC MYCOPLASMA

[75] Inventor: Shyh-Ching Lo, Potomac, Md.

[73] Assignee: American Registry of Pathology, Washington, D.C.

[21] Appl. No.: 710,361

[22] Filed: Jun. 6, 1991

Related U.S. Application Data

[63] Continuation-in-part of Ser. No. 265,920, Nov. 2, 1988, abandoned, which is a continuation-in-part of Ser. No. 875,535, Jun. 18, 1986, abandoned.

[51] Int. Cl.⁵ C12N 5/00; C12N 5/02; C12N 1/00; C12Q 1/70
[52] U.S. Cl. 435/240.2; 435/5; 435/872
[58] Field of Search 435/870, 5, 872, 240.2

[56] References Cited

[57] ABSTRACT

The invention relates to a novel pathogenic mycoplasma isolated from patients with Acquired Immune Deficiency Syndrome (AIDS) and its use in detecting antibodies in sera of AIDS patients, patients with AIDS-related complex (ARC) or patients dying of diseases and symptoms resembling AIDS diseases. The invention further relates to specific DNA sequences, antibodies against the pathogenic mycoplasma, and their use in detecting DNA or antigens of the pathogenic mycoplasma or other genetically and serologically closely related mycoplasmas in infected tissue of patients with AIDS or ARC or patients dying of symptoms resembling AIDS diseases. The invention still further relates to a variety of different forms of vaccine against mycoplasma infection in humans and/or animals.

2 Claims, 39 Drawing Sheets

Similar diseases are transmitted from animal to animal by injecting filtrated lysates of spleen, lymph nodes or whole blood from the diseased animals. *M. fermentans incognitus* is also identified in the cytoplasm of the cytopathic cells. Some of the infected mice were found to produce prominent antibody against *M. fermentans* incognitus.

When silver leaf monkeys are inoculated with *M. fermentans incognitus*, the monkeys show wasting syndromes and die within seven to nine months after inoculation. At necropsy, the monkeys do not show evidence

PUBLICATIONS

Marquart et al (1985) Mycoplasma-Like Structures . . .
Eur J Clin Microbiol 4(1):73-74.

Lo et al (1989) A Novel Virus-like Infectious Agent . . .
Am J Trop Med Hyg 40(2):213-226.

Lo et al (1989) Identification of *M Incognitus* . . . Am. J.
Trop-Med. Hyg 41(5):601-616.

Lo et al (1989) Association of the Virus-like Agent . . .

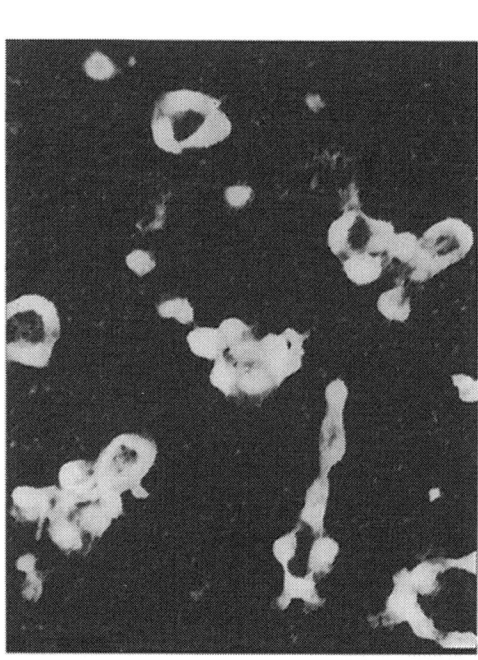

of opportunistic infections, acute inflammatory lesions
35 or malignancy. *M. fermentans incognitus*-specific DNA
can be directly detected in necropsy tissues of the monkeys, by use of polymerase chain reaction method. *M. fermentans incognitus* infection can be identified in
40 spleen tissue, liver tissue, kidney tissue and brain tissue of the monkeys. Some of the infected monkeys produced antibody to *M. fermentans incognitus*.

1. Detection of *M. fermentans incognitus* Antigens

45 The *M. fermentans incognitus* pathogen is useful for the detection of antibodies in the sera of patients or animals infected with *M. fermentans incognitus*. Some of these patients who are infected with *M. fermentans incognitus* will be patients who have been diagnosed as
50 having AIDS or ARC, Chronic Fatigue Syndrome, Wegener's Disease, Sarcoidosis, respiratory distress syndrome, Kibuchi's disease, autoimmune diseases such as Collagen Vascular Disease and Lupus and chronic debilitating diseases such as Alzheimer's Disease. In one
55 procedure, presistently *M. fermentans incognitus* infected cells are grown in low cell density on sterile glass slides. Sera from suspected patients, and normal subjects are examined in an immunoperoxidase staining procedure such as that described by Hsu, S-M., et al.,
60 *Am.J.Clin.Path.* 80, 21 (1983). Using this assay, 23 of 24 sera from AIDS patients showed strong positivity. Serum from the other AIDS patient showed weak posi-

"The Third Time's a Charm"

The following is a quote from the book entitled, *Amyotrophic Lateral Sclerosis* co-written by Donald W. Scott and his son, William L.C. Scott, regarding the filing of the patent:

"On June 18, 1986, representatives of the US Division of Microbiology and Immunology, Department of Infectious and Parasitic Disease Pathology, Armed Forces Institute of Pathology, Washington, DC, went to the US Patent Office and filed for a patent on the 'pathogenic mycoplasma.' However, there were certain flaws in the application and they withdrew it."

In a second attempt:

"On November 2, 1988, the same government agency went back to the Patent Office. Under serial number 265,920, they again asked for a patent on the pathogenic mycoplasma. Once again they had to go back to the drawing board because of flaws in their claim."

The third attempt:

"On June 9, 1991, the same government agency along with government microbiologist Dr. Shy-Ching Lo as the 'inventor' filed a new application for a patent."

According to Donald W. Scott's brilliant research:

"Primary Examiner Christine M Nucker and her assistant D.R. Preston went to work on the patent. Finally, they were satisfied that here indeed was a new 'invention' based upon an ancient microorganism. Patent #5,242,820 was approved on September 7, 1993, awarding all rights and claims to the pathogenic mycoplasma to the US government agency, the American Registry of Pathology."

AUTHOR'S COMMENT

Even though our government recognizes mycoplasma as a disease agent, allopathic doctors are still unaware as to what causes autoimmune diseases, Alzheimer's, cancer(s) and many other mycoplasma infections. The subject of mycoplasma is not taught in allopathic medical schools. Information has been kept secret about mycoplasma for over 100 years.

The Driving Forces behind the Epidemic

Cancer and disease are definitely infections. Dr. Royal Rife in the 1930s proved it. (See Rife Machine chapter.) Many Americans are infected with Lyme disease, mycoplasma, Candida, Chlamydia pneumoniae or other disease-causing pathogens, including viruses.

Many suffer from chronic depression or hormonal imbalance. I believe the following were the "driving forces" behind the worldwide epidemic of cancer and disease:

THE SEXUAL REVOLUTION

By far the "sexual revolution" started the ball rolling and got us where we are today.

Today, "hooking up" is considered the "norm;" but in reality, it is downright dangerous. Sex is not Russian roulette anymore. The more sexual partners your partner has had, the greater at risk <u>you</u> are. You <u>will</u> definitely get infected if you share body fluids with an infected person. Women are at the greatest risk.

Now Lyme disease (see Lyme disease chapter) is being sexually transmitted and has become a worldwide epidemic.

SUGARLAND, USA

Another contributing factor is the main ingredient in the typical American diet--sugar. No matter where we go or what we do, we are bombarded with sugar. All the major holidays encourage the consumption of sugar, i.e., Halloween, Christmas, Thanksgiving, and Easter. All food commercials on TV promote "sugary" products.

Compared to fifty years ago, Americans now have sugar bellies. (Excess sugar calories are converted into fat around the middle.)

FACT: Mycoplasma metabolizes sugar and cannot survive without it. A very low sugar diet will starve it.

Change is in the horizon for Americans who wish to survive this cancer and disease epidemic. (See the ketogenic diet on page 88.)

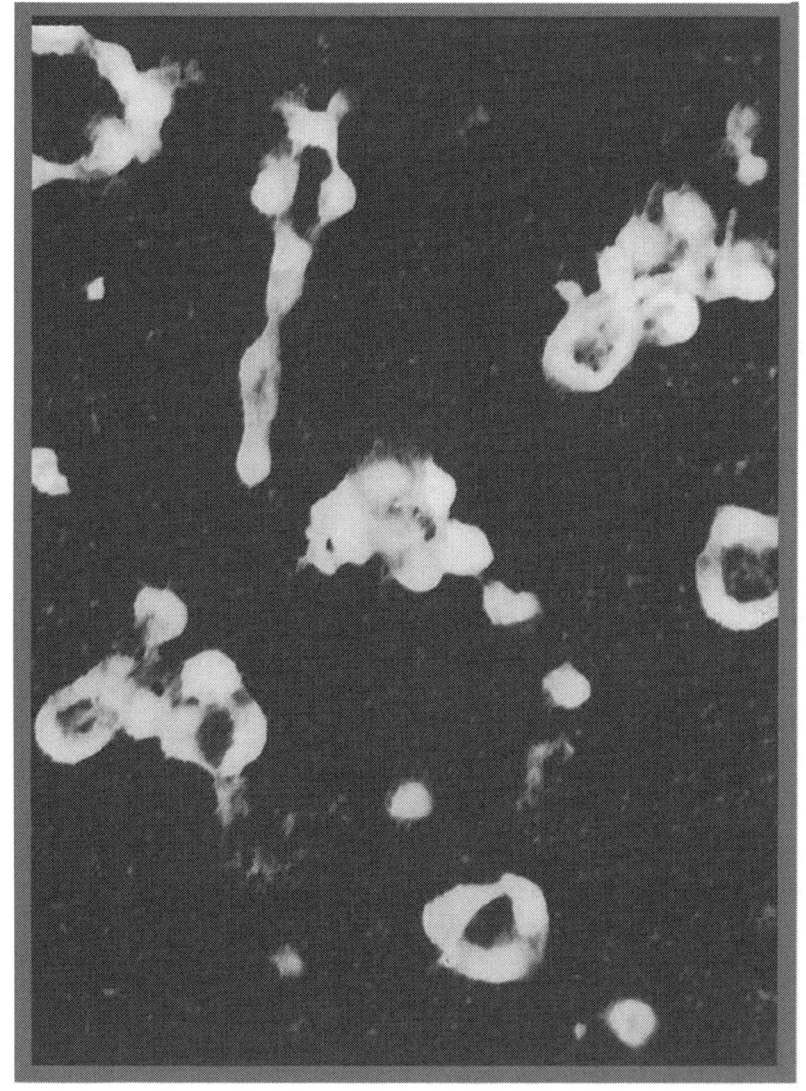

Mycoplasma in various stages of growth. (Provided by Dr.. HaroOld Clark)

Mycoplasma Q&A

Since 2003 when I first learned about mycoplasma, I learned as much as I could about the subject. I have compiled the following:

Q. What is mycoplasma?

A. A mycoplasma (cell wall-deficient bacterium) is the DNA strand of a bacterium. It is encased in a double cell membrane. Since it has no cell wall, it has no organelles. Therefore, it is parasitic in nature. Some mistakenly describe a mycoplasma as a fungus. Some call it a prion. Some scientists mistakenly call it a retrovirus since it resembles the AIDS virus.

Q. Do antibiotics work against mycoplasma?

A. No, because a mycoplasma has no cell wall. Therefore, the body's only natural defense is the immune system, and most of the US population has a dysfunctional or compromised immune system. (See chapter entitled, Mycoplasma, Nagalase and GcMAF, page 52.)

Q. Do doctors know about mycoplasma?

A. To answer this question, we have to go back some 100+ years to the Louis Pasteur days of medicine. There were two opposing sides. Louis Pasteur's theory was that bacteria do not change shape. The opposing side believed that bacteria could change shape (pheomorphism) according to the environment, i.e., they can change to rods or shed their cell wall.

Unfortunately, for us, allopathic medicine chose Pasteur's theory. Therefore, mycoplasmas do not exist in the eyes of allopathic medicine. Obviously, allopathic medicine had to come up with an explanation for the cause of disease/cancer.

They adopted the "autoimmune theory," which implies "the immune system is attacking the body." Using steroids, they treat the disease and/or cancer by "shutting off" the immune system, which stops the immune response (symptoms). This is by far "Dark Ages" medicine. No functioning immune system means mycoplasmas can spread to other organs and tissue (metastasize).

FYI: According to the book *The Cancer Cure that Worked*, on his deathbed, Louis Pasteur confessed he was wrong.

NOTE: If the truth ever came out that cancer and disease are infections and that there are safe effective treatments that kill pathogens, the current medical/industrial complex would collapse.

Q. Is mycoplasma contagious and how is it spread?

A. Yes. Health care workers and caregivers of infected patients are at the greatest risk. A mycoplasma is the smallest living organism. It can cross the blood-brain barrier. It can also be found in body fluids (mouth, mucus, spit, seminal fluid, etc.) and can even be transmitted from one person to another through sex and breathing recycled air on airplanes. (Wearing a surgical mask is useless.)

Q. If mycoplasma is contagious, why isn't everyone sick?

A. Most everyone *IS* infected—asthma, rheumatoid arthritis or cancer, for example. Even symptom-free people have mycoplasma lying dormant inside a degenerative cell. It is just waiting for an opportune time to awaken.

Q. What awakens it?

A. Usually a trauma awakens mycoplasmas. The trauma can be emotional or physical. For example, it could be a car accident, a fall, a reaction to bad surgery, a rape, a divorce, the loss of a job, a loved one being sick, the loss of a loved one, and so on. Mycoplasmas also awaken if the host is experiencing long bouts of extreme stress, as in a stressful job situation.

Q. Why trauma or stress?

A. The answer lies in the host's pH. To stay healthy, a human cell must be in a state of alkalinity (~7.25-7.45). Most bacteria (there are exceptions) and viruses are the opposite. They thrive in an acidic environment (bacteria 5-6.8). When we experience a trauma or extreme stress, our bodies become acidic. If their environment suddenly changes and becomes acidic (a jolt to the system), mycoplasmas will activate.

For a more detailed explanation, read the chapters entitled It's No Acident Why Some People Do Not Get Sick, page 65.

Q. What are the symptoms of a mycoplasma infection?

A. Chronic fatigue, brain fog, lack of balance, depression, granulomas (boils) under the arms, low grade fevers, neuropathy, joint pain, nerve damage, migraine headaches, loss of libido, hormonal imbalance, just to name a few.

Q. What are some diseases and cancers caused by mycoplasma?

A. See the Mycoplasma Literature chapter, page 28.

Q. I have a mycoplasma infection. Why am I so depressed?

A. Mycoplasmas cause hormonal imbalance. Mycoplasmas need cholesterol (cell membrane) to replicate. The easiest place for a mycoplasma to find cholesterol is in the endocrine system, where hormones are produced. Cholesterol is one of the main components of a hormone. Eample: We need hormones (endorphins) to keep from being depressed.

Q. I have a mycoplasma infection. I can't sleep. Why?

A. Again, we need hormones to help us sleep.

Hormones regulate body temperature (hypothalamus) and this is why some infected people cannot regulate body temperature. It is the same for the loss of libido (thyroid gland).

Q. Why is chronic fatigue associated with a mycoplasma infection?

A. First, the cell is defenseless on the inside. (The immune system is on the outside.) Inside the host cell, the mycoplasma is parasitic, using the cell's internal cell components to replicate.

The damaged cell eventually dies and ruptures, spilling out the newly replicated mycoplasmas, along with the contents of the cell. According to mycoplasma researchers, one of the amino acids inside the cell is glutamate.

Glutamate is an "excitotoxin" and causes nerve cells to "fire." When glutamate is outside the cell, this triggers a chemical reaction. The body turns glutamate into glutamine (they are in the same family). The process to turn glutamate into glutamine is as follows:

CONVERTING GLUTAMATE TO GLUTAMINE

To convert glutamate into glutamine, the body takes an ammonia ion off of urea in the bloodstream, causing the release of a cyanide ion. The cyanide ion then enters a neighboring cell where it focuses on the battery of the cell (mitochondria). At the fourth complex of the mitochondria Kreb's cycle, the cyanide uptakes the energy generated. This deprives the cell of its energy and results in the (temporary) shutdown of that cell, resulting in chronic fatigue.

The cyanide does not kill the cell. According to researchers, red blood cells neutralize cyanide.

Q. Is air rage associated and caused by mycoplasma?

A. Mycoplasmas flare up in a change in barometric pressure such as on an airplane.

FYI: The movie star Rita Hayworth (diagnosed with Alzheimer's) went berserk during a flight and was taken off the plane in a straightjacket.

Q. What about altitude sickness?

A. Since mycoplasmas are anaerobic, they do not use oxygen. High altitude means less oxygen. It is very common for mycoplasmas to flare up and become even more aggressive/active in high altitude.

One night I was watching a movie on TCM (cable TV). It is customary for the movie host to tell a little trivia about the star of the movie before the movie begins. The following story is a perfect example of mycoplasmas flaring up in high altitude:

Rosalind Russell, a well-known movie star in the 1930s, was diagnosed with breast cancer. She was offered a movie role to be shot on location in the mountains. She accepted; but during the filming of the picture, she was diagnosed with rheumatoid arthritis. Aggressively, because of the high altitude (low oxygen) the mycoplasma spread (metastasized) from her breasts to her joints.

Q. Will there ever by a cure for cancer or disease?

A. The word "cure" is misleading. The answer is "no," there will never be <u>permanent</u> immunity, a cure or a vaccination for cancer or disease. Cancer and disease are infections. Effective treatments kill disease - causing pathogens, but <u>a person can get re-infected</u>.

Q. What is the Herxheimer reaction?

A. When mycoplasmas die, they release endotoxins (cell membrane), which trigger an immune response.

Depending on the severity of the immune response to toxins released by microorganisms in the bloodstream, the host may experience chills, fever, aches and pains, vomiting, etc. When fighting the flu, you are actually experiencing a Herxheimer's reaction.

Mycoplasma's outer membrane is made up of lipopolysaccharides, classified as endotoxins. Endotoxins excite and activate the immune system's white blood cells. I think of it this way: An endotoxin is to a mycoplasma as a drop of blood is to a shark. This then causes a "feeding" frenzy. (See Venus flytrap chapter.)

Q. If researchers call AIDS a virus, why do you call it a mycoplasma?

A. AIDS virus is not a "true" virus. AIDS was invented (created in a lab), which explains why a US patent could be issued. It might be one of the first GMO's. AIDS is a cell wall-deficient bacterium with the genetic material of the Visna virus (mad cow disease) and is vulnerable to the same treatments that kill mycoplasmas.

Q. On the subject of viruses, are there effective ways to kill a virus?

A. Yes, Goldenseal in this book, page 147.

Q. Do mycoplasmas attack damaged cells?

A. Damaged tissue is weak. You will recognize the movie star in the following story:

He was the representative for a very large soda company in his early years. According to his autobiography, he drank 24 cans of diet soda every day. (As just about everyone knows, Aspartame is a neurotoxin and damages brain cells.)

I do not know the circumstances as to what triggered Parkinson's disease in this movie star, but it is easily explained why he came down with Parkinson's. Something triggered the mycoplasmas to awaken in his brain, which attacked his "damaged" brain cells. He is now the spokesperson for the Parkinson's Foundation.

This story may convince you to stop drinking soft drinks, which are extremely acidic—one to three on the pH scale. (See Section 2 – "Balancing".)

Q. Can animals get mycoplasma infections?

A. Yes, they can get diabetes, cancer, and diseases, too. Some of the protocols in this book (especially mild silver protein) can be used on animals.

Symptoms of a Mycoplasma Infection

Much of what I have learned about mycoplasma is from the Common Cause Medical Research Foundation's journal(s). If not for the courageous work of its founder, Donald W. Scott (died on December 6, 2011), this world would be a much "darker" place to live. I owe my health and my life to both Dr. Harold Clark and Donald W. Scott.

The following are typical symptoms of a mycoplasma infection, whether it presents as cancer or disease:

- Chronic fatigue
- Fibromyalgia
- Chronic headaches and bouts of nausea
- Hyper sensitivity to temperature and barometric changes
- Cognitive problems, i.e., "brain fog"
- Short-term memory loss
- Emotional imbalance (bi-polar or depression)
- Endocrine system (hormonal) imbalance
- Reproductive system problems (infertility), which may include loss of libido, endometriosis, and spontaneous abortion
- Granulomas under the armpits
- Frequent bouts of generalized pain
- Reduced blood volume
- Gout (not in ALL cases)

According to researchers, mycoplasmas can exist in an inert (inactive) form called a crystal or they can convert to a liquid state under certain conditions of pressure, temperature, and pH.

There are 100+ species of mycoplasmas--ten found in humans. According to researchers, mycoplasmas derived from the bacteria brucellia abortus DNA are referred to as mycoplasma fermentans incognito. Mycoplasma fermentans causes fibromyalgia, bi-polar depression, Alzheimer's, Parkinson's, ALS, and many other auto-immune diseases and cancers. (The Brucellosis bacteria can attack ANY and ALL systems in the body.)

According to research, mycoplasma wreaks havoc in the endocrine system (where the body makes hormones), i.e., causing dysfunction in the hypothalamic, pituitary, adrenal, pancreas, and thyroid as follows:

Cholesterol is one of the pre-formed sterols that mycoplasma uptakes for replication. Cholesterol is an essential prerequisite to the generation of hormones necessary to the maintenance of the body's metabolic balance. The sequence is:

$$\text{co-enzyme} + \text{squalene} + \text{cholesterol} = \text{hormone}$$

If this sequence is disrupted by a mycoplasma's uptake of cholesterol, the production of various hormones is interfered with, as is the case of the hypothalamic regulation of sleep or body temperature. When this happens, irregular sleep patterns and extreme sensitivity to temperature occurs.

Mycoplasma Literature

The following appeared in a 2004 edition of The Journal of Degenerative Diseases, Vol 5, No. 4:

Human diseases and conditions that are caused by mycoplasmas, or where mycoplasmas are a key co-factor therein:

AIDS ([1 ch 3], 2, 3, 4, 5, 6, 7, 8, 13, 21, 22, [51 p 4-12]), ARC (7), Arthritis (1, 16, 17, 21, 31), Alzheimer's (7, 14), asthma (13, 14, 16, 31), ALS (13, 14, 50), adrenal failure (7), acute stem cell leukemia (33), abnormal liver function (31), acute glomerulonephritis (31), acute psychosis (17), aggressive cancers (14), arterial sclerosis (51), apoptosis (22), altered lymphocyte responses (5), autoimmune reaction (27, 36), abscess (29), ascending paralysis (31), arthalgias (7, 31), anklosing spondylitis (54), Bullous myringitis (17, 24, 29), brain stem encephalitis (31, 41), breast cancer (61), Chronic Fatigue Syndrome (7, 9, 13, 14, 21, 50, [51 p 4-12], 55), Chronic lymphocytic leukemia (38), cardiac complications (1 p. 421), collagen vascular disease (7 47, 56), Creuzfeldt-Jakob (51 p.12), congestive heart failure (31), Crohn's (14, 21), conjunctivitis (7, 17, 31), chromosome aberrations (21, 30, 49), cerebellar ataxia (31), central nervous system disease (1, 7, 17,21), CNS in infants (25, 31), chronic cystitis (1 ch 25, p. 431), cardio vascular disease (14, 21), confusion (7), CSF infection (25), congenital pneumonia (23), chronic bronchitis (31), chronic pulmonary disease (31), cranial nerve palsies (31), chorioamnionitis (31), cervical adenopathy (40), Diabetes mellitus (14, 50), dysplasia (18), death ([1 ch 27 p465], [1 ch 32 p539], 17, 31), Endometriosis (1 ch 25 p 431), erythematous macula papular and vesicular exanthemas (21, 31), endocarditis (13, 50), epididymitis ([1 ch 25 430], 31)erytherma nodosum (17), erytherma multiforma minor (17), Fibromyalgia (9, 13, 14, [51 p 35-36], 55), facial neuropathy (51 p 19-26), Gulf War Illness (13, 14, 21, 50, [51 p 4-12]), Guillain Barre (17, 31), Graves Disease (13, 15), glomerulosclerosis (7), gangrene (31), gastrointestinal symptoms ([1 p421],31), Huntington's (51), Hashimoto's thyroiditis (15), hemolytic anemia (17, 31), hemiplegia (1), heart failure (7), hypercalcemia (7), hemopericardium (31), hypogamma-globulinemia (1 ch 25 pp 421, 427, 431), hepatitis (31), hydrocephalus ([1 ch 25 p431], 25), hypoxemia (31), hemogluinuria (31), hyercoagulability (31), Inflammatory bowel disease (13, 14, 46), infertility ([1 p426], 19, 31, 32, 56), immune system damage (6, 21), interstitial cystitis (14), intravascular co-agulation (31, 50), idiopathic Thrombocytopenia purpura (33), joint infection (1 ch 25 p427), juvenile chronic arthritis (54), Kawasaki (15), Kibuchi's Disease (7), kidney stones (20), lupus (7, 12, 13, 14, 15, 29, 39, 51, 52, 56), low birth weight ([1 ch 25 p431], 56), leukemia ([1 ch 29 p 498], 14, 21, 28, 33, 34, 35, 38), lymphoma (14), liver (21, 7), lung abscess (38), lympho sarcoma (38), lymphadenopathy (7), leukopenia (3), lymphopenia (3), Meningo encephalitis (17, 31) myocarditis (13, 16, 31, 50), malignant transformation (21), multiple sclerosis (13, 14, 15, 50), multiple organ failure (50), meningitis ([1 ch 25 p 427 & 431], 16, 31), myalgia (7, 31), macular rashes (31), mordaleiform rashes (31), Nongonccal urethritis ([1 ch 25 p428], 26, 29, 31), non- Hodgkin's lymphoma (21), nervous system infection of neonates (1 ch 25 p 431), neural lesions (31, 41), neo-natal morbidity (56), nasal polyps (45), neurological complications (1 ch 25 p 421), Oncogenic transformation (49), otitis medial ([1 ch 25 p 421], 17), otitis externa (17), primary atypical pneumonia ((([1 ch 25 p 428], 7, 13, 14, 16, 17, 21, 23, 24, 27, 29, 36, 40), pelvic inflammatory disease ([1 ch 25 p 426], 14, 31), pancreatitis (31), psychosis (31) Pharyngitis ([1 ch 25 p 421], 17, 21, 27, 29, 40), pyelonephritis ([1 ch 25 p 426], 31), post partum fever (31), proteinuria (7), pityriasis rosea (31), psoriatic arthyritis (54), Parkinson's disease (51), polyarteritis of brain and heart (31), prostate cancer (60), prostatitis ([1 ch 25 p 430], 26, 31), polyarthritis ([1 ch 25 p 427 & 431], 31), pericarditis (13, 31, 50), psoriasis (14, 51), pleural effusion (31), peteceal rashes, papulo vesicular rashes (31), respiratory distress syndrome ([1 ch 25 p 427 & 537], 31, 50), rheumatoid arthritis ([1 ch 25 p 435, ch 29 p 498], 12, 13, 14, 21, 29, 39, 53, 54, 56), Reiter's([1 ch 25 p 431], 29, 31, 39), rheumatic fever (17), respiratory disease in newborns ([1 ch 25 p 431], 23), renal failure (7, 31), red blood cell alteration (27, 42), Raynaud's disease (31, 51), reactive arthritis (54), Sarcoidosis (7, 51), Sjogren's Syndrome (14, 15), scleroderma (11, 12, 14), Steven's Johnson Syndrome (17, 31, 51), spontaneous abortion ([1 ch 25 p 431], 28, 31), suppurative arthritis (1 ch 25 p 427 & 431), septicemia ([1 ch 25 p 421 & 427], 29), solid cancers(14), Swyer Jones Syndrome (31), subcutaneous abscess ([1 ch 25 p 431], 31), stillbirth ([1 ch 25 p 431], 23, 31), scaly erythema (31), submandublar adenitis (3), transverse myelitis (10, 31), tracheo bronchitis (1 ch 25 p 418 & 421, 17, 21, 23, 27, 36), thrombocytopenia (8, 31), ulcerative stomatitis (31, 46), urethritis (26), uriticaria (1), vaginitis (1 ch 25 p 426), Varicella-like rashes (31), vasculitis (14), Wagener's (7).

MYCOPLASMA DISEASES IN ANIMALS

(Includes dogs, cats, cows, horses, sheep, goats, pigs, rodents, gorillas, elephants, seals, buffalo, elk, mule deer, crocodiles, tortoises, chickens, turkeys, geese, falcons, vultures, and insects.)

Arthritis (17,47), abortion (17), abcess (23), alopecia (7), acute neurological syndrome (47), adreno cortical activation (48), brain lesions (41,47), behavioral alterations (48), contagious bovine and caprine pleuropneumonia (17), contagious agalectia (17), chronic progressive polyarthritis (47), cachexia (17), dehydration (17), death (7,17,41,47), distended capillaries (4,10), Encephalopathy (47), edema (7,17,41), fibrinoid necrosis (47), fatal systemic infection in primates (7), fibrosis (47), genital disorders (17), immune dysfunction (7), Kerato conjunctivitis (7), leukemia (1 pp 599-605), leukopenia (7), leukocytosis (7), lymphocyte depletion (7), mastitis (17), neurological disorders (7, 41), neuroendocrine alterations (48), ocular disorders (17), pneumonia (17), perivascular round cell infiltration (23,47), poly arteritis (17,47), paralysis (7), rolling disease (1 Ch 27 p 463,41), respiratory disease (17,47), rhinitis (17), synovial membrane hypertrophy (47), Spongiform Encephalopathy (41), skin lesions (17), thromboses in lymphs, arteries and veins (23), vessel sclerosis (47), vesicular lesions (41)

1. Mycoplasmas: Molecular Biology and Pathogenesis - J. Maniloff, Editor-in-Chief, 1992, American Society for Microbiology ISBN 1-55581-050-0

2. A Novel-like Infectious Agent in Patients with AIDS - S. Lo, et al. American Journal of Tropical Medicine and Hygiene 40(2) 1989, pp. 213-226 (8-246)

3. A Fatal Injection of Silvered Leaf Monkeys with a Virus-like Infectious Agent (VLIA) Derived from a Patient with AIDS - S. Lo, et al. American Journal of Tropical Medicine and Hygiene 40(4) 1989, pp. 399-409 (8-350)

4. Association of the Virus-like Infectious Agent Originally Reported in Patients with AIDS with Acute Fatal Disease in Previously Healthy non-AIDS Patients - S. Lo, et al. American Journal of Tropical Medicine and Hygiene 41(3) 1989, pp. 364-376 (9-098)

5. Virus-like Infectious Agent (VLIA) is a Novel Pathogenic Mycoplasma: Mycoplasma Incognitus - S. Lo, et al. American Journal of Tropical Medicine and Hygiene 41(5) 1989, pp. 586-600 (89-163)

6. Identification of Mycoplasma Incognitus Infection in Patients with AIDS: An Immunohistochemical in situ Hybridization and Ultrastructure Study - S. Lo, et al. American Journal of Tropical Medicine and Hygiene 41(5), pp. 601-616 (89-164)

7. Mycoplasma Fermentans (Incognitus Strain) Infection in the Kidneys of Patients with Acquired Immune Deficiency Syndrome and Associated Neuropathy - F. Bauer, et al. Human Pathology, Jan. 1991 Vol. 22 No. 1, pp. 63-69

8. US Patent # 5,242,820 Pathogenic Mycoplasma, Lo

9. Thrombocytopenia Purpura in Patients with Acquired Immunodeficiency Syndrome Related Complex - J. Nair, et al. Annals of Internal Medicine 1988, 109, pp. 209-212 UI: 88267631

10. Examinations of Mycoplasmas in Blood of 565 Chronic Illness Patients by Polymerase Chain Reaction - M. Nasrella, et al. International Journal of Medicine, Biology of the Environment 2000, 28(1), pp. 15-23

11. Transverse Myelitis Associated with Mycoplasma Pneumoniae Infection - M. Ablehorn, et al. Clinical Infectious Diseases April 1998 26:4, pp. 909-912

12. Scleroderma - The Proven Therapy That Can Save Your Life - Henry Scammel, Road Back Foundation

13. Road Back Foundation Newsletter, Fall 2000

14. Mycoplasmal Infections in Chronic Illnesses: Fibromyalgia, Gulf War Illness, HIV-AIDS, and Rheumatic Arthritis - G. Nicolson, et al. Medical Sentinel, Vol. 4, No. 5, Sept/Oct 1999, pp. 172-175

15. Mycoplasmas: The Missing Link in Fatiguing Illnesses - M. Guthrie. Alternative Medicine Sept 2001, Issue 43 pp. 60-70

16. The Pathogenesis and Treatment of Mycoplasmal Infections - G. Nicolson, et al. Antimicrobics and Infectious Diseases Newsletter Nov 1998, Vol. 17, No. 11, pp. 81-87

17. Studies Suggest a Darker Side of Benign Microbes - J. Stephenson. JAMA Dec. 17, 1997, Vol. 278, No. 23, p. 205(2)

18. Methods in Molecular Biology: Mycoplasma Protocols - Editor Roger Miles and Robin Nicholas, (Human Press)

19. Mycoplasmas & Dysplasia of the Uterine Cervix - R. Averan, et al. Boll. 1 Siertor Milan st 1980, Sept 30, 59(4), pp. 348-358

20. Mycoplasma, Chlamydia, Epstein-Barr, herpes I and II, and AIDS Infections Among 100 Consecutive Infertile Female Patients and Husbands: Diagnosis, Treatment and Results - R. B. Knudson, et al. International Journal of Fertility, Nov-Dec 1986, 31(5), pp. 356-359

21. Mirkin Report: Why I Prescribe Antibiotics - Gabe Mirkin, MD., P.O. Box 10, Kensington, MD 20895 (extensive references)

22. Mycoplasmas: Sophisticated, Reemerging and Burdened by Their Notoriety - J. Baseman and J. Tully. Emerging Infectious Diseases 1997, Vol. 3, No.1

23. Links and Interactions Between Mycoplasmas and Viruses: Past Confusions and Present Realities - C. Chastel Arch. Virol 1995 140 pp. 811-826

24. The Mycoplasmas Vol. 14 Mycoplasma Pathogenicity - S. Razin and M.F. Barile, Editor, pp. 65-106

25. Epidemiology of Mycoplasma Pneumonia Infection in Families - H. Foy, et al. JAMA Sep 12, 96, Vol.197, #11, pp. 859-865 (137-143)

26. Ureaplasma and Mycoplasma Infections in the Central Nervous System of Preterm Infants- N.J. Shaw, et al. The Lancet Dec 23/30, 1989, pp. 1530-1531

27. Recovery of Pleuropneumonia-like Organisms from Negro Men with and Without Nongonoccal Urethritis - M. Shepherd. American Journal of Syphilis, Gonorrhea, and Venereal Diseases 1954, Vol. 38, pp. 113-124

28. Mycoplasma Pneumoniae Infections in Volunteers - C. Smith and R. Chanock. Annals of NY Academy of Sciences 1967, Vol.m143, pp. 113-124

29. Isolation and Identification of Mycoplasma from Human Clinical Materials - L. Hayflick and & Stanbridge. Annals of NY Academy of Sciences July 28, 1967, No. 1, pp. 608-621

30. Human Mycoplasma Infections - M. C. Shepherd. Health Laboratory Science, Washington- American Public Health Association July 1966, Vol. 3, No. 3 H.L.S., pp. 163-169

31. Chromosome Changes in Humans Diploid Cell Cultures Infected with Mycoplasmas - G. Patton, et al. Nature July 3, 1965, Vol. 207, pp. 43-45

32. Mycoplasmas as Agents of Human Disease - G. Cassell and B. Cole. The New England Journal of Medicine, 1981, June 8, Vol. 304, No. 2, pp. 8-89

33. Serological Evidence that Chlamydia and Mycoplasmas are Involved in Infertility of Women - B.R. Moller, et al. Journal of Reproduction and Fertility, 1985, Vol. 73, pp. 237-240

34. Virus Studies of Human Leukemia - W. Murphy, et al. Cancer 1965, Vol. 18, No. 10, pp. 1329-1344

35. Isolation of Mycoplasma from Leukemic and Nonleukemic Patients - W. Murphy, et al. Journal of the National Cancer Institute, Aug 1970, Vol. 45, No. 2, pp. 243-251

36. Direct Isolation of Mycoplasmas from Human Leukemiic Bone Marrow - L. Hayflick and H. Kaprowski. Nature Feb 13, 1965 Vol. 205 pp. 713-714

37. The Mycoplasmas. Mycoplasma Pathogenicity Vol. IV, Barile, Immunizations Against Mycoplasma Infections 1985, Academic Press, pp. 452-481

38. The Molecular Biology of Mycoplasma Viruses - J.Maniloff & A. Liss. Annals of NY Academy of Sciences 1973, Vol. 225, pp. 149-158

39. Mycoplasmas (PPLO) and Human Leukemia and Lymphoma - J. Grace, et al. Cancer 1965, Vol. 18, No. 10, pp. 1369-1379

40. Isolation of Mycoplasma (PPLO) from Patients with Rheumatoid Arthritis, Systemic Lupus Eryematosus and Reiter's Syndrome - L. Bartholomew & J. Himes. Arthritis and Rheumatism, 1964, Vol. 7, pp. 291-end

41. Exudative Pharyngitis Following Experimental Mycoplasma Hominis Type I Infection - M. Murfson, et al. JAMA June 28, 1965, Vol. 192,No. 13, pp.1146-1152

42. Studies of PPLO Infection III, Electron Microscopic Study of Brain Lesions Caused by Mycoplasma Neurolyticum Toxin - D. Aleu and L. Thomas. The Journal of Experimental Medicine Volume 124, 1966, pp. 1068-1082

43. Studies of PPLO Infection II, The Neurotoxin of Mycoplasma Neurolyticum - L. Thomas, et al. Journal of Experimental Medicine 1966, Vol. 124, pp. 1068-1082

44. Mycoplasma Pneumoniae Infections in Volunteers - C. Smith and R. Chanock. The Annals of the NY Academy of Sciences 1967, Vol. 143

45. Human Spongiform Encephalopathy: The Nat'l Institute of Health Series of 300 Cases of Experimentally Transmitted Diseases - P. Brow, D.C. Gajdusek. Annals of Neurology 1994, Vol. 35, No. 5, pp. 513-528

46. Infectious Amyloids: Subacute Spongiform Encephalopathies as Transmissible Cerebral Amyloidosis - D.C. Gajdusek. Fields of Virology, Third Edition, (Chapter 91) 1996, pp.2851- 2900

47. The Detection of Mycoplasma Pneumoniae in Nasal Polyps - P. Garr, et al. Clinical Otolaryngology, 6/1996, 21:3, pp.269-273

48. A Prospective Study of Viral and Mycoplasmal Infections in Chronic inflammatory Bowel disease - Kangro, et al. Gastroenterology 1990, Vol. 98, pp. 549-553

49. Pathogenesis Studies in Experimental Mycoplasma Disease - W. Clyde & L. Thomas. Annals of the NY Academy of Sciences 1973, Vol. 225

50. The Role of Brain Cytokines in Mediating the Behavioral and Neuroendocrine Effects of Intra Cerebral Mycoplasma Fermentans - R. Yirmiya, et al. Brain Res. 1999, May 22; 829 (1-2), pp. 28-38

51. Mycoplasmas and Oncogenesis: Persistent Infection and Multistage Malignant Transformation - L. Tsai, et al. Proclamation of National Academy of Sciences, USA, Oct. 24, 1995, 92(22), pp. 10197-10201

52. Through the Looking Glass: A Country Doctor's Journey in the Labyrinth of Gulf War Syndrome - L. Goss. International Journal of Medicine, Winter 1998, No.s 2, 3 & 4, pp. 10-16

53. Journal of Degenerative Diseases - Donald W. Scott, Editor. Feb 2002, Vol. 3, Nos. 3 & 4

54. Mycoplasma Urealyticum and Mycoplasma Hominis in Women with Systemic Lupus Erythematosus - K.S. Ginsburg, et al. Arthritis and Rheumatism 1992, 33, pp. 429-433 55. Detection of Mycoplasma Antigens in Immune Complexes from Rheumatoid Arthritis Synovial Fluids - H. Clark, et al. Ann. Of Allergy 1988, 60, pp. 394-398

56. Identification of Mycoplasma Fermentans in Synovial Fluids Samples from Arthritis Patients with Inflammatory Disease - S. Johnson, et al. Journal of Clinical Microbiology, Jan. 2000, 38(1), pp. 90-93

57. Fibromyalgia, Chronic Fatigue Syndrome, and Myofacial Pain Syndrome - D. Buskilia. Current Opinions in Rheumatology March 2000, 12(2), pp. 113-123

58. The Potential Roles of Mycoplasma as Autoantigens and Immune Complexes in Chronic Vascular Pathogenesis - H. Clark. American Journal of Primatology 1991, 24, pp. 235-243

59. Antibiotics for Huntington's Disease? - Science News, Aug. 19, 2000, Vol. 158, p. 120

60. Persistent Exposure to Mycoplasma Induces Malignant Transformation of Human Prostate Cells - Kazunori Namiki, et al, Sep 1, 2009

61. Pleomorphic mammalian tumor-derived bacteria self-organize as multicellular mammalian eukaryotic-like organisms; morphogenetic properties in vitro, possible origins, and possible roles in mammalian 'tumor ecologies', by Douglas H. Robinson, April 16, 2004

More Facts about Mycoplasma

The following is a quote from page 119 of *The Brucellosis Triangle* <u>co-written</u> by Donald W. Scott and his son, William L.C. Scott. (He is referring to the weaponized Brucellosis bacterial mycoplasma:

> "Incorporated into the bacteria from which the bacterial toxin* is extracted and crystallized is a human herpes virus related to Epstein-Barr or to HIV-6. This element contributes to the damage by reducing the body's immune system capacity to cope with the toxin."

*Toxin denotes mycoplasma/nucleus

THE SLEEPING MYCOPLASMA

When a "host" first becomes infected with mycoplasma, this is what happens, according to *The Burcesllosis Triangle*, page 119:

> "The bacterial toxin* works by linking to a gene in the cell's DNA or in the cell's mitochondria. There it will lie relatively passive until some trauma triggers its nucleating process. The useless protein fibril** generated will either kill the cell or disable it by destroying the ability of the mitochondria to provide the cell with its energy."

*Toxin denotes mycoplasma

**Fibril denotes amyloids

AMYLOIDS

Donald W. Scott describes mycoplasma as a particle, an amyloid, a prion, and/or a virion. The following is from *The Brucellosis Triangle*, page 104-105 describing mycoplasma:

> "It is a sub-viral particle which lacks a nucleic acid and hence is incapable of reproducing itself. However, if it invades a cell in the brain of a genetically predisposed subject, this particle (variously called an amyloid, a prion, virion or other) will begin a process of protein fibril formation. These useless fibrils grow to occupy and kill the cell leaving it as part of the sclera or scar."

According to mycoplasma researchers, mycoplasmas can invade the mitochondria and attack the mitochondria's DNA, thus shutting it down leaving the cell with no energy.

If these fibrils (mycoplasmas) are released into the bloodstream, they will invade other healthy cells and destroy them, too.

ALZHEIMER'S

When cells are killed in the brain by mycoplasmas, this leaves lesions, which interfere with the chemical processes of the brain. According to *The Brucellosis Triangle*, page 122:

> "These lesions are etiologic in the decreased regional cerebral blood flow found in Alzheimer's."

PARKINSON'S

If mycoplasmas attack a host in the occipital lobe of the brain, the victim is diagnosed with Parkinson's. The occipital lobe is directly connected to the optic nerves and to the eyeballs. This part of the brain is in "intimate contact" with the limbic system, which produces substances that allow the brain to function.

SCHIZOPHRENIA AND MULTIPLE SCLEROSIS

The following is a quote from *The Brucellosis Triangle*, page 105:

> "Schizophrenia, like MS, is caused by brain scarring, principally in the medial temporal lobe areas. Such lesions can produce symptoms of inappropriate emotional response to external stimuli, severely interrupting social interactions, i.e., the victim is 'mentally ill.' Or if the lesions are only slightly removed from the medial temporal lobe areas to the ventricular areas, the victim is afflicted with multiple sclerosis."

FIBROMYALGIA AND GOUT

Again, the following is a quote from *The Brucellosis Triangle*, page 71:

> "Gout is caused by an excess of uric acid crystals usually found in the joint of the big toe. The excess uric acid may be due to the digestion of rich foods in nucleic acids such as liver, kidneys and other ofals. This is the high-living disease associated with Henry VIII. Or the excess of uric acids may be due to the breakdown of nucleic acids in the body cells.
>
> Amyloids caused from brucellosis replicate themselves within selected cells and in the process liberate the damaged cell's nucleic acid. When the released nucleic acid breaks down into

uric acid, it forms into crystals which cause the pain of gout and arthritis."

Further, when uric acid crystallizes and is deposited in certain muscle masses and joints, this produces excruciating pain associated with fibromyalgia.

MYCOPLASMA AND KIDNEY FAILURE

When the nucleic acid from the dead cells is released into the bloodstream, the body turns these nucleic acids into uric acid. These, in turn, crystallize and when the kidneys cannot handle the volume of uric acid, hyperuricemia occurs. This could lead to kidney stones. Further, uric acid crystals can obstruct the kidney's interstitium and tubules leading to kidney failure and death.

My father suffered with Parkinson's for over 20 years. He did not die of Parkinson's. He died from kidney failure.

Anemia and Mycoplasma

All life forms need iron. Bacteria use iron in co-enzymes and DNA synthesis (replication). Over time, bacteria have developed mechanisms for the intake of iron when their environment is not hospitable. The following are the stages of how bacteria (mycoplasmas, for example) cause chronic anemia in humans. (For your convenience, definitions are at the end of this chapter.)

Stage 1

Bacteria (mycoplasma) invade cells. The infected cells release cytokines (chemical distress signals) and the first to appear on the scene are phagocytic neutrophils.

Next to arrive are macrophages. Inflammatory cytokines are released and inflammation (plasma) surrounds the "infected" tissue. More and more macrophages arrive at the site.

NOTE: Macrophages are responsible for engulfing and killing pathogens and repairing damaged tissue. They convert arginine to nitro oxide if they are fighting pathogens. For tissue repair, they convert arginine into ornithine.

Macrophages are also the "cleanup crew." They recycle iron when they "eat" and dispose of red blood cells at the end of the red blood cells' life cycle (~120 days). Especially important, macrophages become the "keepers of the iron" and are responsible for releasing iron to newly manufactured red blood cells.

Stage 2

As inflammation increases due to the release of more cytokines and the inflammation increases, the liver starts releasing hepcidin, a hormone, which <u>inhibits</u> macrophages from releasing iron into the bloodstream. (This is a built-in safeguard to keep bacteria from accessing iron. Making iron scarce slows down bacterial growth. However, over time, this negatively affects the host.)

Stage 3

An increase in inflammation causes the bone marrow to produce more white blood cells instead of red blood cells.

Due to the macrophages holding onto iron internally, newly created red blood cells are <u>not</u> receiving sufficient amounts of iron, which enables hemoglobin to transport oxygen to the now oxygen-starved cells. Symptoms of anemia begin to show up in the host.

Bacteria secrete siderophores and steal iron from the hemoglobin and the plasma. As the infection worsens, chronic anemia manifests. Ultimately, less and less oxygen is getting to the cells, even though there are sufficient amounts of iron in storage. (Less oxygen in the body causes mycoplasma to aggressively speed up even more.)

Stage 4

Suffering from chronic anemia, the host's heart is now overworked, as it is forced to pump harder and harder to get more oxygen to the cells. This could lead to death--congestive heart failure. Cancer patients and the elderly are especially vulnerable.

AUTHOR'S COMMENTS

According to sources, blood transfusions are not the answer. "New" blood makes iron readily available to mycoplasmas, which enable them to flourish and replicate even faster.

Definitions

Anaerobic Respiration is used by bacteria, which do not use oxygen to make energy. Instead of using oxygen, anaerobic bacteria (mycoplasmas) use sulfate, nitrate, sulfur, or fumarate as electron acceptors, which manufacture far less ATP's (energy) than aerobic respiration.

Anemia is usually defined in three ways: (1) as a decrease in the amount of red blood cells in the blood; (2) the decreased amount of hemoglobin in the blood; or (3) a lowered ability of the blood to carry oxygen. Symptoms of anemia are tiredness, weakness, feeling faint, shortness of breath, or an inability (strength) to exercise.

Blood Plasma is the pale yellow liquid component of blood, which holds the blood cells in suspension. Plasma makes up 55% of the body's total blood volume. It consists of 95% water and contains dissolved proteins, glucose, electrolytes, clotting factors, hormones and CO_2.

Cytokines define a category of small proteins, which are important in cell signaling. All cells with a nucleus produce cytokines.

Ferroportin is a trans-membrane protein that transports iron from the inside of a cell (macrophages, for example) to the outside of the cell. It is inhibited by hepcidin. Therefore, iron is not transported out of the cells. It is kept internalized.

<u>Hemoglobin</u> is an iron-containing oxygen-transport protein found in red blood cells and macrophages. It needs iron to carry oxygen.

<u>Hepcidin</u> is a hormone produced in the liver, which reduces dietary iron absorption. Inflammation and the release of cytokines trigger the liver to release hepcidin. Hepcidin, in turn, inhibits ferroportin by binding to it and keeps it and iron inside macrophages, the main site of iron storage. Hepcidin also reduces iron absorption through the gut and reduces iron exit from the liver.

<u>Inflammation</u> is the initial bodily response to harmful stimuli, which results in the increased movement of plasma and leukocytes (WBC) to the affected site.

<u>Iron</u>, a potentially toxic substance, is important to human health and disease. Iron is a highly electrical acceptor/receptor and is used to attract and carry oxygen to cells. Because it is so toxic by itself, life forms use proteins to bind and carry iron. If left free, iron catalyzes hydrogen peroxide into free radicals, which can damage the cell and kill it. Macrophages break down and process old red blood cells. They recycle and store most of the iron in the body. (NOTE: Iron is very important in the Vitamin C IV Therapy chapter, page 186.)

<u>Leukocytes</u> are white blood cells (WBC) of the immune system, used by the body to fight disease-causing pathogens. Used to repair the body, white blood cells are produced in the bone marrow (stem cells). Five types of leukocytes exist, including monocytes and netrophils, which are phagocytic (kill pathogens). An increase in the number of WBC's in the blood is an indicator of infection.

<u>Macrophages</u> are a type of evolved monocytes (WBC), which are detrimental in the healing process, removing debris and dying cells in the blood, and killing pathogens. When it "retires" a "spent" red blood cell by engulfing it, it then acts as an iron-storage container. Later, it releases iron to newly formed red blood cells. FYI: Macrophages can "eat" and digest up to 100 pathogens in its lifetime (120 days).

<u>Neutrophil</u> are a type of leukocyte and are phagocytic. They are the first immune system cells to appear at an injured site or the site of an infection.

<u>Red Blood Cells</u> (RBC) lack a cell nucleus to accommodate more room for hemoglobin. FYI: 2.4 million new red blood cells are produced

every second in human adults. They develop in the bone marrow and circulate 100-120 days, after which they are recycled by macrophages. It takes a red blood cell only 20 seconds to travel a full circle in the human body. One-fourth of the cells in the body are red blood cells. They are the principle carrier of oxygen to the tissues. RBC's are very flexible and when squeezing through capillaries, release oxygen to the cells.

Siderophores are small, iron-chelating compounds secreted by bacteria and fungi to absorb iron. They are amongst the strongest soluble binding (electrical acceptors) agents known to science. After releasing siderophores to "catch" iron, bacteria reabsorb them, along with the captured iron.

Nitric Oxide

Nitric oxide (NO) is a gas molecule that has a life of just a few seconds. Nitric oxide is manufactured in the endothelium, which is the inner most lining of blood vessels. Endothelium is only one cell thick; therefore, it cannot be seen by the naked eye.

When the smooth muscles surrounding the blood vessels constrict, nerve stimulation prompts the endothelium to synthesize (manufacture) and release small amounts of nitric oxide, which relax the muscles.

When the endothelium is healthy and producing nitric oxide, the endothelium is as smooth as Teflon. When it is not producing and releasing nitric oxide, the endothelial cells become "sticky" and become vulnerable to bacterial plaque formation.

Nitric oxide:

- Eliminates inflammation in the blood vessels associated with plaque
- Inhibits the formation of plaque in the blood vessels
- Most importantly, <u>dilates</u> and <u>relaxes</u> blood vessels, increasing blood flow

In the documentary, *Forks Over Knives*, patients with heart disease who stayed on a plant-based diet reversed their heart disease. This mystery as to how and why they could reverse high blood pressure, diabetes and heart disease is explained in a forthcoming chapter (see The Truth about Enzymes chapter, page 194).

AUTHOR'S COMMENTS

Cardiovascular disease is the #1 cause of death in the United States. Even after the discovery of nitric oxide in 1998, the "real" cause of heart disease is still a mystery to medical researchers.

After researching and reading about nitric oxide, a Pandora's Box opened and the connection between cardiovascular disease and pathogenic microorganisms was no longer a mystery.

The following is from "The Journal of Degenerative Diseases," entitled The Media…Mass Murder…and Modern Medicine, Spring/Summer, 2003, Volume 4, Number 2&3:

> "Researchers have recently been able to culture *C. pneumoniae from obstructive atherosclerotic lesions. C. pneumoniae, hiding in the arterial plaque in structures of

foam-cell fatty matter that it builds around itself, takes years (often decades) to kill the infected person. This allows multiple opportunities for the 'symptom-free' person to pass the infection to others through respiratory secretions during cold or flu season."

*C. pneumoniae = Chlamydia pneumoniae (a bacterium)

The next chapters explain the connection between bacteria and heart disease in the following sequence:

> (1) Mycoplasma, Nitric Oxide and ADMA
>
> (2) The Truth about Heart Disease

Mycoplasma, Nitric Oxide and ADMA

The human body is relatively a bag of chemicals and chemical reactions. If something directly or indirectly disrupts or stops the body from functioning and/or processing chemicals, the affected cells/tissues in the body shut down or dysfunction.

Arginine

Arginine is an amino acid that is in the Glutamate family. (Family members include glutamate, glutamine, proline and arginine.) Most importantly, the Glutamate family is the <u>source</u> (especially glutamate and glutamine) for forming nitrogen groups in the cells.

Arginine plays an important role in:

- Cell division
- Healing wounds and bones
- Removing ammonia from the body
- Immune defense (killing of pathogens)
- The release of hormones

Another important point is the immune system and endothelial cells turn arginine into nitric oxide (NO).

Nitric Oxide (NO)

As part of an immune response, phagocyts produce nitric oxide.

According to Wikipedia:

> "Nitric oxide is secreted as free radicals in an immune response and is toxic to bacteria and intracellular parasites, including Leishmania and malaria."

Mycoplasmas attack a cell and wreak havoc, taking what they need to replicate. Eventually the cell dies, and ruptures, spilling out the contents of the cell, along with the replicated mycoplasmas. Note: In the contents of the cell is the amino acid glutamate.

According to mycoplasma researchers, the body cannot tolerate "free roaming" glutamate and turns glutamate into glutamine. This is "<u>protein modification,</u>" (the protein glutamate modified into glutamine).

According to allopathic researchers, "protein modification" in the body causes the production of ADMA.

Asymmetric dimethylarginine (ADMA)

According to Wikipedia, the following is a description of Asymmetric dimethylarginine (ADMA):

> "ADMA is a naturally occurring chemical found in the blood plasma. It is a metabolic product of <u>continual protein</u> modification processes in the cytoplasm of all human cells."

Scientists do not understand what is causing "protein modification" in the body. However, they do know that ADMA inhibits the endothelial cells from turning arginine into nitric oxide, but they cannot explain why. (ADMA is a marker in the blood for heart disease.)

Here is the sequence:

Mycoplasma infection ☐Cell death ☐Protein modification (glutamate to glutamine) ☐ADMA is produced ☐ADMA inhibits the production of nitric oxide ☐ Dysfunction of endothelial cells (unable to dilate and relax blood vessels) ☐ Cardiovascular Disease (high blood pressure, "sticky" blood vessels, hardening of the arteries) ☐ Plaque buildup ☐ Heart attack/stroke ☐Death.

DID YOU KNOW?

There are over 100,000 miles of blood vessels in the human body?

Erectile dysfunction is the first clinical indication of cardiovascular disease.

The Truth about Heart Disease

From the previous chapter, a mycoplasma infection indirectly causes the inhibition of the production of nitric oxide (NO), which then causes the endothelial cells to become "sticky," which leads to the formation of arterial plaque (biofilm).

Biofilm

"Birds of a feather flock together"

According to Wikipedia:

> "Biofilms have been found to be involved in a wide variety of microbial infections in the body, by one estimate 80 percent of all infections."

What is biofilm? Inside biofilms are colonies of microorganisms; i.e., bacteria, archaea, protozoa, fungi, and algae. In this chapter, bacterial biofilm, particularly Chlamydia Pneumoniae plaque, is the focus. Bacteria colonize for protection. The following are the four stages to form a biofilm colony:

Stage One: Bacteria attach to the host's "sticky" endothelial cells.

Stage Two: More and more bacteria arrive, including mycoplasma, which adhere to the host.

Stage Three: The biofilm colony grows as the bacteria use the host's cells to replicate.

NOTE: C. Pneumoniae and mycoplasma are parasitic and rely on the host to furnish "material" to replicate.

FACT: The outside protective wall of the biofilm is built by bacteria and has many layers consisting of polysaccharides, lipoproteins, lipids, minerals, and other debris, either secreted by the bacteria or from the outside (bloodstream).

Biofilms are not entirely flat. The biofilm takes on a vertical structure, which allows the biofilm colony to "catch" and take in nutrients from outside the biofilm environment. This structure (see diagram, page 49) is designed to allow the release of byproducts more easily.

The multiple layers of the biofilm protect the bacteria from the immune system, besides keeping essential enzymes inside to keep them in close proximity to the colony.

Stage Four: The biofilm ruptures and bacteria disperse (metastasize) to establish new colonies. C. pneumoniae leave the colony to travel to the lungs to exit and be transferred to other hosts through the secretion of body fluids (cold and flu).

DID YOU KNOW?

Biofilms can harbor other pathogens such as fungus (mold and yeast). They can all live under the same "roof," parasitically sharing and/or competing for the same nutrients.

According to Wikipedia:

"Infection processes in which biofilms have been implicated include common problems such as urinary tract infections, catheter infections, middle-ear infections, formation of dental plaque, gingivitis, coating contact lenses, infections in cystic fibrosis, and infections in devices such as joint prostheses and heart valves."

Biofilm's surface has the same electrical charge (negative) as the immune system's cells. This is why the immune system at first ignores the colony. Once the plaque is in place, the immune system has a tough time breaking through the biofilm to reach the pathogens.

DID YOU KNOW?

Scientists and doctors blame macrophages for lesions in arterial plaque, which lead to a heart attack or stroke.

The following "break down" or penetrate biofilm:

- Lactoferin (see Colostrum chapter)
- Ozone
- Pancreatic Enzymes (see Enzyme Therapy chapter)
- DMSO (see Sulfur chapter)
- Vitamin C therapy

FYI: Plaque, mycoplasma fibrils (amyloids), along with C. pneumoniae have been found in the brains of autopsied Alzheimer's victims, are still puzzling allopathic medical doctors and researchers.

Bacterial Plaque

Stages 1 & 2
Free-floating mycoplasma (using pili) attach to host tissues. More mycoplasma join. Using cell-to-cell communication, they form a colony by using pili to bind to each other and to their host.

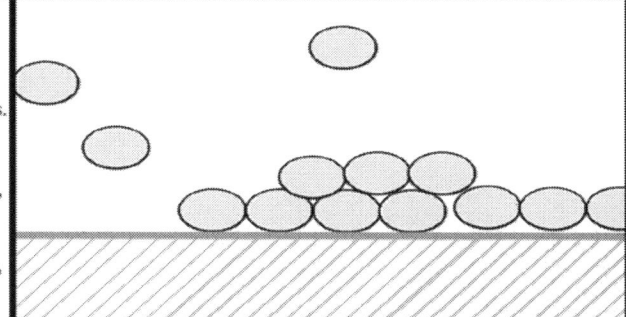

Stage 3
Bacteria build a biofilm protecting themselves from the immune system. Biofilm is made from protein, fat, sugar, minerals and debris either secreted or from the host. Biofilm keeps enzymes inside. Space between the two towers collects free-floating minerals in the bloodstream for bacteria.

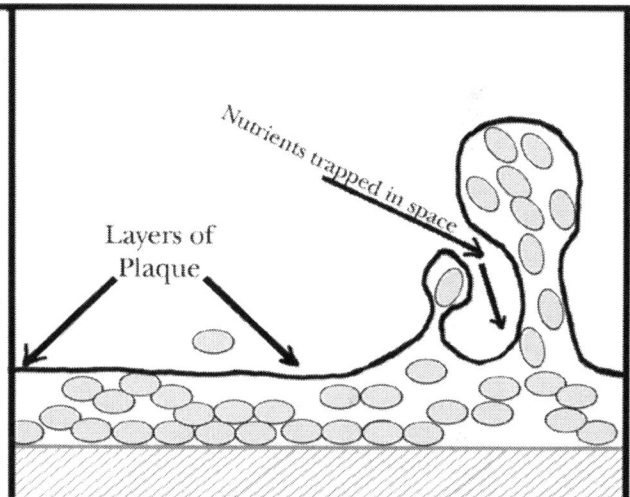

Stage 4
Mycoplasma can cohabitate with other bacteria (Chlamydia pneumoniae). Mycoplasma can leave the colony to form new colonies and the infection spreads to other tissues or organis (metastasizes)

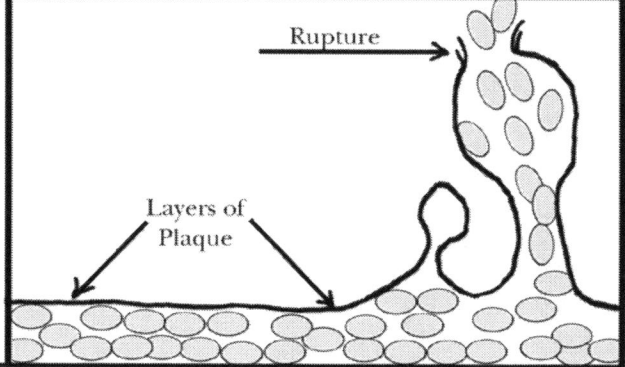

Mycoplasma and the Cachexia Cycle

One-half of all cancer patients suffer from cachexia. Wikipedia defines cachexia as a "wasting syndrome."

According to other sources, this is one of the leading causes of death in cancer patients, autoimmune diseases (Parkinson's and Alzheimer's), and AIDS victims.

It's a vicious circle--the cachexia cycle. When the cancer cell (mycoplasma) ferments sugar into lactic acid, the lactic acid ends up in the blood stream, where it travels to the liver where it is converted right back into glucose which goes right back to the cancer cell (mycoplasma) and feeds it again. This cycle keeps endlessly repeating and repeating.

In the meantime, the lactic acid is blocking the healthy cells from getting nutrients. Everything is going to and feeding the mycoplasmas in the cancer cells. Eventually, the patient's muscles and tissue begin breaking down as the body starts "wasting away."

AUTHOR'S COMMENTS

Have you ever seen Alzheimer's in the final stages? The victim is "wasting away" (cachexia cycle). The victim's joints are "fixed" in the fetal position, while the body is literally being starved to death and reduced to a bag of skin, organs and bones.

Hydrazine Sulfate ($H_6N_2O_4S$)

There is a very sad story behind the development and medical industry's refusal to use hydrazine sulfate, and cancer patients are the ultimate victims.

In the 1970s, Dr. Joseph Gold designed hydrazine sulfate specifically to address cachexia. Here's how hydrazine sulfate works:

When the liver converts lactic acid back into glucose, it requires an enzyme (phosphoenolpyruvate carboxykinase a/k/a/ PEP CK) to process the lactic acid. Hydrazine sulfate <u>blocks</u> this enzyme and, therefore, lactic acid is not converted back into glucose. (And you can imagine the rest.)

In studies Dr. Gold showed that in 50 percent of cancerous lab animals, the animals started gaining their weight back. In his studies, "tumors began to shrink."

DID YOU KNOW?

Hydrazine sulfate causes cancer cells to starve and die!

It has not been banned or is not illegal to use hydrazine sulfate, however, it should only be administered through an alternative medical professional.

Hydrazine sulfate cannot be taken with alcohol, tranquilizers, sleeping pills, and foods containing the amino acid breakdown product tyramine (aged cheeses, raisins, avocados, processed fish and meats and other fermented products).

Mycoplasma, Nagalase and GcMAF

NAGALASE

Enzymes are essential. According to Wikipedia:

> "Enzymes are known to catalzye more than 5,000 biological reaction types. Almost all metabolic processes in the cell need enzymes."

Mycoplasmas produce the enzyme N-acetyl-Galactosaminidase (nagalase) to break down large sugar molecules, specifically N-acetyl-Galactosamine.

THE IMMUNE SYSTEM

Macrophages are the "Pac-Mans" of the immune system. What do they do? They attack and destroy pathogens. They signal other immune cells of an invader by leaving parts of the pathogen's carcass behind (called an antigen). They are also the "cleanup" crew.

If macrophages are out of commission—the entire immune system is compromised, and infection (disease/cancer) *WILL* inevitably occur or spread (metastasize).

Basically, macrophages are "sleepy" creatures, but when the host is threatened or being attacked by pathogens—they are activated. What triggers and activates macrophages? Answer: GcMAF

GcMAF

GcMAF is an acronym, Globulin Compound-derived Protein Macrophage Activating Factor. GcMAF consists of a modified GC protein (the transporter) and vitamin D. The following is a simplified explanation.

There are several steps the body must take to produce GcMAF:

Step 1: The liver converts plasma protein into Gc-Protein. NOTE: At this stage, the Gc-Protein has a sugar side chain consisting of <u>three</u> sugar molecules – a tri-saccharide [triple sugar]:

- N-acetyl-Galactosamine
- Galactose
- Sialic Acid

Step 2: For the GC protein to become a Macrophage Activating Factor and be able to transport vitamin D, two of the sugar molecules (galactose and sialic acid) must be stripped away. Galactose is removed by the enzyme beta-galactosidase, which is embedded in the outer cell membrane of a B-lymphocyte. Sialic acid is removed by the enzyme sialidase, which is located in the outer membrane of a T-lymphocyte.

Step 3: Once stripped of the two sugar molecules, the GC protein is ready to become GcMAF. NOTE: In all my research (many hours) it was unclear where and when vitamin D binds with the stripped down GC protein, but once it bonds with the GC protein, it becomes GcMAF.

GcMAF then "wakes up" a dormant macrophage by attaching to the macrophage's outer cell receptor. This signals the macrophage to become cytotoxic (to hunt down and kill pathogens).

Step 4: One macrophage can destroy many pathogens and "eat" cancerous tumor cells (mycoplasmas are inside the cancer cells). It then leaves pathogenic debris (antigens) behind, which activates and signals other immune cells to get busy.

MYCOPLASAMA INFECTION

Enzymes always do what they are supposed to do. No exceptions. When the "host" has a mycoplasma infection, mycoplasmas release nagalase into the bloodstream where the enzyme encounters N-acetyl-Galactosamine attached to the GC protein. Instantly, nagalase strips the sugar molecule (N-acetyl-Galactosamine) from the GC protein. This then blocks vitamin D from attaching to the GC protein. It's that simple.

NOTE: It does not matter when nagalase comes into contact with the GC protein, i.e., before, during or after the other two sugars are removed by the T or B- lymphocytes. The end product is not GcMAF. The striped-down GC protein becomes a useless protein.

Now the host is in danger. He or she has no immune response. The dormant macrophages are unaware of what is going on and the entire immune system is compromised.

As the infection spreads, more and more nagalase is being released—blocking GCMAF from being produced.

THE IMPORTANCE OF VITAMIN D

Direct sunlight on the face, arms and legs for at least 5 to 30 minutes twice a week is needed to produce enough vitamin D to stay healthy. The darker the skin, the more minutes it takes for the skin to make vitamin D. In the case of too much sun exposure, excess Vitamin D biodegrades.

Vitamin D is needed to absorb calcium in the gut. Insufficient amounts of Vitamin D causes osteoporosis and rickets (softened bones). Vitamin D is needed to absorb minerals.

FYI: Sunscreen blocks the skin from making Vitamin D.

According to experts, if you must take a vitamin D3 supplement, make sure it is not synthetic.

DID YOU KNOW?

The presence of nagalase in the blood is a cancer marker.

Mycoplasma and Vaccines

Even ten years ago, mycoplasma researchers knew that vaccines were contaminated with mycoplasma. It is impossible to filter out mycoplasma, the smallest living organism. Mycoplasmas can also attach to cell walls in cultures and escape detection.

Dr. Bradstreet, an autism researcher/doctor, was murdered in 2015, possibly because he had discovered unusually high levels of nagalase and mycoplasmas in his autistic patients' blood. (For verification, watch and listen to Dr. Bradstreet speaking at autism conferences on youTube.)

Dr. Bradstreet was treating his autistic patients <u>successfully</u> with GcMAF, until government(s) around the world shut down labs producing GcMAF.

It is now illegal in the US to possess, buy, sell or manufacture GcMAF.

AUTHOR'S COMMENT

As far as I know, the only country where doctors are allowed to use GcMAF is Japan.

VACCINES

The following is typically in a vaccine:

- Ethylene glycol (anti-freeze)
- Phenol/carbolic acid (used as a disinfectant/dye)
- Formaldehyde (known to cause cancer)
- Aluminum (used to promote antibody response)
- Thimerosal (mercury disinfectant/preservative)

Vaccines are grown in animal or human tissue (aborted fetuses). This could possibly be the reason why people develop allergies to certain animals. (The immune system makes antibodies against "foreign" substances in the vaccine.)

AUTHOR'S COMMENTS

I recommend watching the movie *Vaxxed*. The movie's theme is about the relationship between the MMR vaccine and autism. FYI: One in eight Americans has autism.

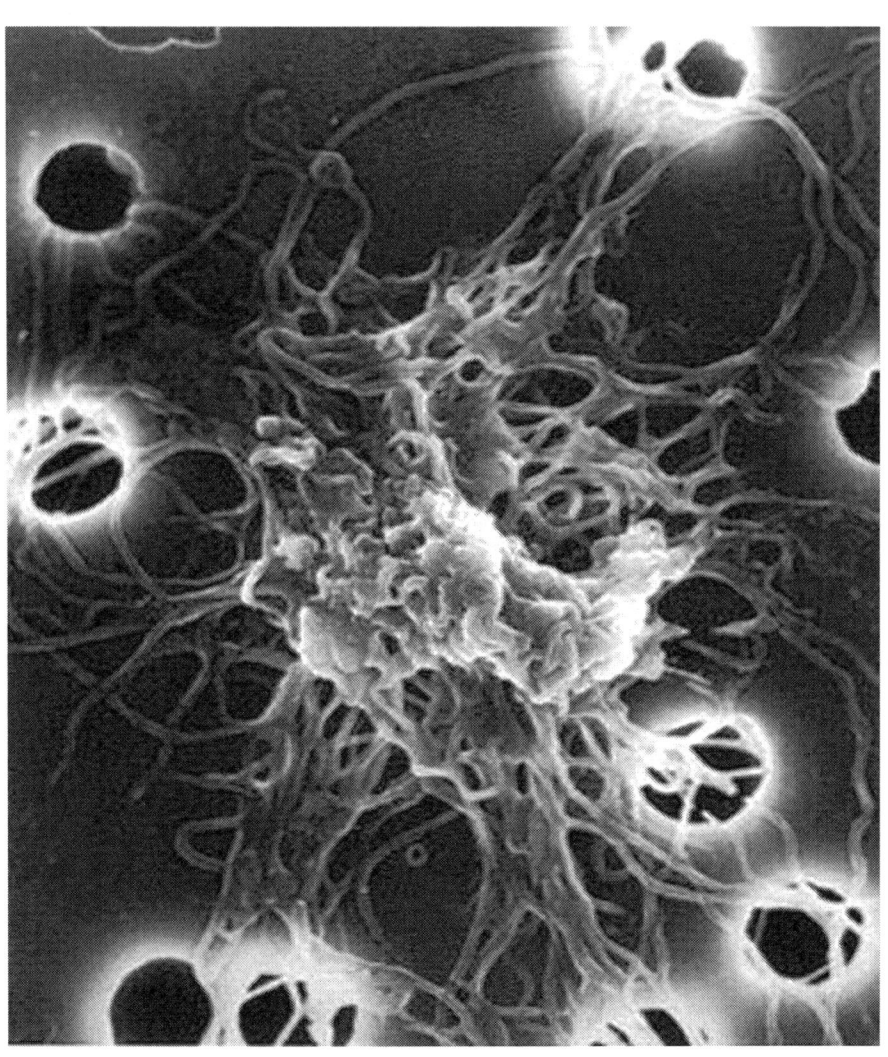

Lyme Disease

Spirochaetes (pronounced spy-row-keets) are an order of double-membraned bacterium, which have corkscrew-shaped bodies (cells). (FYI: The corkscrew shape helps them penetrate and bore into tissue.)

Most of them are aerobic, with a few exceptions. Lyme spirochaetes use manganese for metabolism and are encased in a membrane (no cell wall). This makes them resistant to antibiotics, but it also makes them vulnerable to certain protocols, especially mild silver protein, page 182.

Spirochaetes differ from mycoplasmas. Their outer membrane has multiple flagella, which allows them to move about.

NOTE: Flagella are appendages used to propel an organism. Example: A sperm cell uses its flagellum to propel itself through the female reproductive tract.)

There are three families within the order (Brachyspiraceae, Leptospiraceaeu, and Spirochaetaceae). Some of the pathogenic spirochaetes are:

Leptospira Species

There are ten different types of Leptospira that cause disease in humans. Leptospirosis, also known as rat catcher's fever, is caught from animals, especially rodents. Leptospirosis is transmitted by infected animal urine that comes into contact with openings in the skin, i.e., the eyes, the mouth or vagina. Symptoms are headaches, muscle pain, fevers, bleeding from the lungs, and meningitis.

DID YOU KNOW?

The optimal pH for the growth of this spirochaete is 7.2-7.6 (alkaline). This spirochaete is "extracellular," meaning it generally lives on the outside of the host's cells. Since they are in the same order, the borrelia spirochaete (Lyme disease) can live in an alkaline pH, too.

Treponema pallidum

This subfamily of spirochaetes causes syphilis, which, if left untreated, causes death. Not until the 1940s, when penicillin (antibiotics) was introduced was syphilis treatable.

The following are notables who had syphilis: Casanova, Al Capone, Napoleon Bonaparte, Vincent van Gogh, Adolph Hitler, Howard Hughes, and Benito Mussolini.

The next spirochaete has spread around the world and is becoming an epidemic. Left untreated, it attacks the joints, central nervous system, organs, and brain and causes a horrible painful death.

Borrelia bergdorferi (Lyme disease)

The first case of a disease with arthritic-like symptoms was observed in 1975 in Lyme, Connecticut.

In 1977, the deer tick was linked to the transmission of this disease, but it was not until 1981 when Willy Burgdorferi discovered the disease was caused by the spirochaetes Borrelia bergdorferi, Borrelia afzelii and Borrelia garinii.

Because the infection first appeared in Lyme, Connecticut, that became its name--Lyme disease.

Since then, researchers have concluded that 12 out of 36 known species of Borrelia cause Lyme disease; but the most prevalent are Borrelia bergdorferi, Borrelia afzelii and Borrelia garinii.

Borrelia spirochaetes are unique. A borrelia spirochaete has a corkscrew shape and is propelled by flagella on <u>each end</u>. (The bacterium is able to move forward by rotating in place.)

This organism can maneuver through gel-like liquid tissue (connective tissue), which enables it to escape the immune system.

FYI: It also releases toxins when it dies, triggering a Herxheimer's reaction.

According to sources, Borrelia spirochaetes use glucose as their primary energy source. They are primarily aerobic but can live in an anaerobic environment.

Typically, Lyme disease is transmitted to humans through the tick bite of a hard-shelled tick known as the deer tick. The following are stages of a deer tick's life, which take about two years to complete the cycle:

Stage 1 - Larvae

Before winter, the infected adult female tick lays up to 3,000 fertilized eggs on the ground. In the spring, the eggs hatch and larvae emerge. Larvae, too, need a host to reach the next stage of development.

Larvae generally latch onto small mammals (rodents) or birds. After feeding (blood), they fall to the ground, molt and become nymphs (tiny immature ticks)

NOTE: Scientists theorize that larvae are infected when feeding on infected hosts, such as birds or the white-footed mouse; after which the spirochaetes become residents in the larva's digestive tract.

(I, myself, believe the larvae are already infected before birth from the mother tick.)

Stage 2 - Nymphs

Nymphs are tiny ticks, which are not ready to mate. They are only interested in one thing--finding a food source. This is the stage where they transfer the borrelia spirochaete to their host, i.e., humans, deer, dogs, and other mammals.

INFECTION

The following is from Microbewiki and explains how the tick transfers Lyme disease to its host:

> "The disease is transmitted to humans from a tick bite when the bacteria migrate up to the tick's salivary glands and through the opening created by the tick. Ticks increase salivation during gorging, prompting the migration of the saliva from the digestive tract. Because migration from the gut takes a few days, transmission of the disease usually does not happen until after the first 24 hours of attachment."

Stage 3 -- Adults

The nymph gorges on blood, molts and becomes an adult. (Sources are unclear as to where the nymphs molt and become adults. Do they stay on the same host, molt, mate and then drop off and lay eggs?) Here's a clue: Sources do emphatically state male ticks <u>are on the host</u>, along with females. The male is not interested in feeding--he is only interested in reproducing.

Logically, this proves a nymph must molt, become an adult, and <u>stay on the host</u> to rendezvous with a "horny" male tick. Otherwise, the sequence would be: molt, drop off the host, become an adult, and then jump back onto the host to encounter a male.

After the fertilization of the female's eggs, she drops off the host and lays the eggs on the ground, at which time another cycle begins.

Springtime is tick season, when nymphs are aggressively searching for a host.

Symptoms

Usually, but not all the time, the first symptoms are a "bull's eye rash, which is visible one to two weeks after the tick bite. The rash lasts three to five weeks. This is when the spirochaete has only infected the skin area of the victim. If treated at this stage, there are no negative complications.

More symptoms can appear along with the rash, such as joint pain, chills, fever and fatigue. Later symptoms include tingling or numbness in the extremities, severe chronic fatigue, severe headaches, chronic arthritis, migraines. seizures, inflammation of joints, and cardiac abnormalities (carditis--inflammation of the heart).

Like its cousin that causes syphilis, it can cross the blood brain barrier and attack brain tissue, causing seizures, migraines, nerve damage, and death.

Testing is very difficult because of the organism's stealth (hiding). Today, standard antibiotics such as doxycycline and amoxicillin are used to treat Lyme disease.

AUTHOR'S COMMENTS

Lyme disease has similar symptoms of a mycoplasma infection. Typically, when the immune system is compromised or overwhelmed by one pathogen, other pathogens join in and the host ends up with multiple infections (co-infections).

DID YOU KNOW?

Dr. Alan MacDonald, MD was the first to discover spirochaete biofilm. He is a researcher featured in the documentary, *Under Our Skin*, which is on youTube.

The spirochaete attaches to collagen where the immune system is unable to reach it.

When first bitten by a tick use castor oil packs on the area. Wrap in gauze. Castor oil is anti-microbial and helps heal the wound. (See Castor Oil chapter, page 163.)

Section 2

"Balancing"
the
Cells

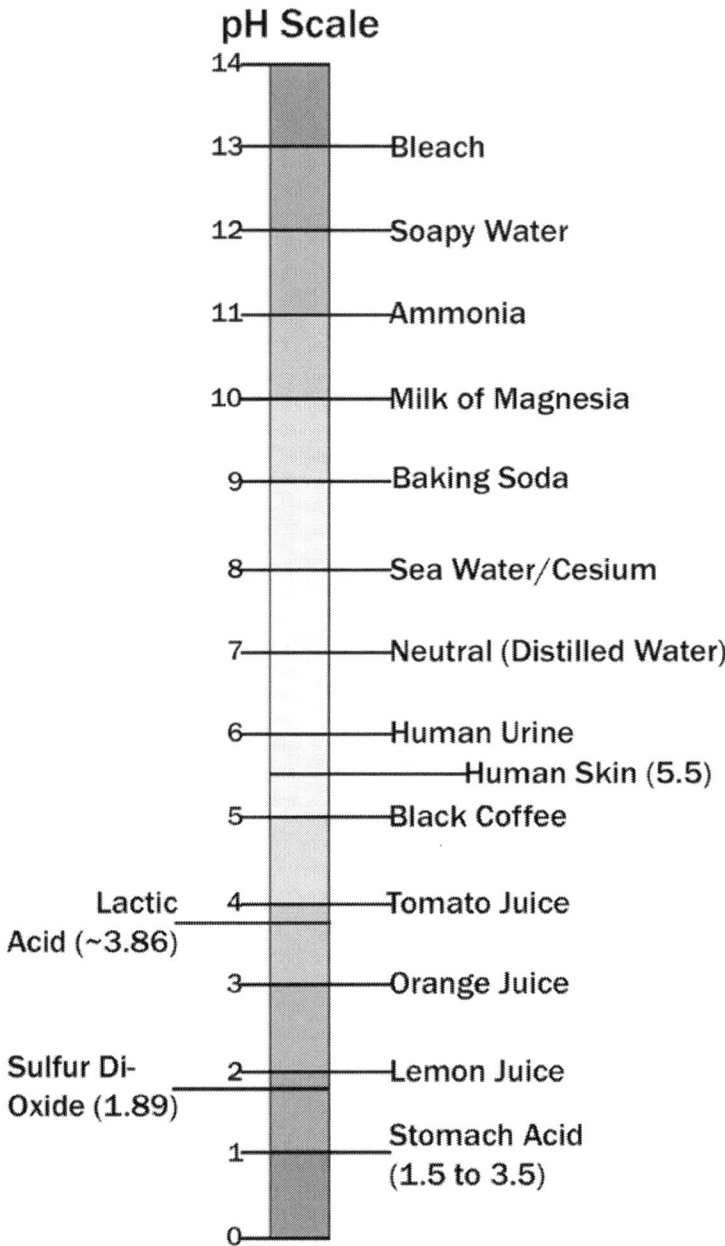

Introduction

Alkaline/Acid pH

To understand "why," it is important to know that microorganisms are the opposite of mammals. Most microorganisms do not flourish in an alkaline environment. They flourish and thrive in an acidic environment. (See next page.)

The gut is to humans as the soil is to plants, meaning the pH of both the gut and the soil has to be acidic to accommodate the "friendly" bacteria, which break down/compost food.

Unfriendly Bacteria

Disease-causing bacteria (mycoplasmas, for example) are unfriendly bacteria. They are anaerobic, the opposite of friendly aerobic bacteria. It is very important that mammals maintain an alkaline pH everywhere in the body except the gut. Otherwise, the unfriendly bacteria can colonize in "unbalanced" degenerative or damaged cells in the body. Cancer and/or disease will then manifest.

Normally, the host's "friendly" bacteria kill the "unfriendly" bacteria in the gut; and if the host's immune system is functioning, the immune system will also kill the unfriendly bacteria.

Author's Comments

Even if you use the protocols in this book to kill mycoplasma, unless your body's cells are "balanced" (alkaline pH), the chances are you will get infected or re-infected by "unfriendly" bacteria.

It is all about maintaining "balanced" cells--a pH of 7.25 to 7.45. This will discourage bacteria and yeast (Candida) from colonizing where they are not supposed to be.

pH Scale

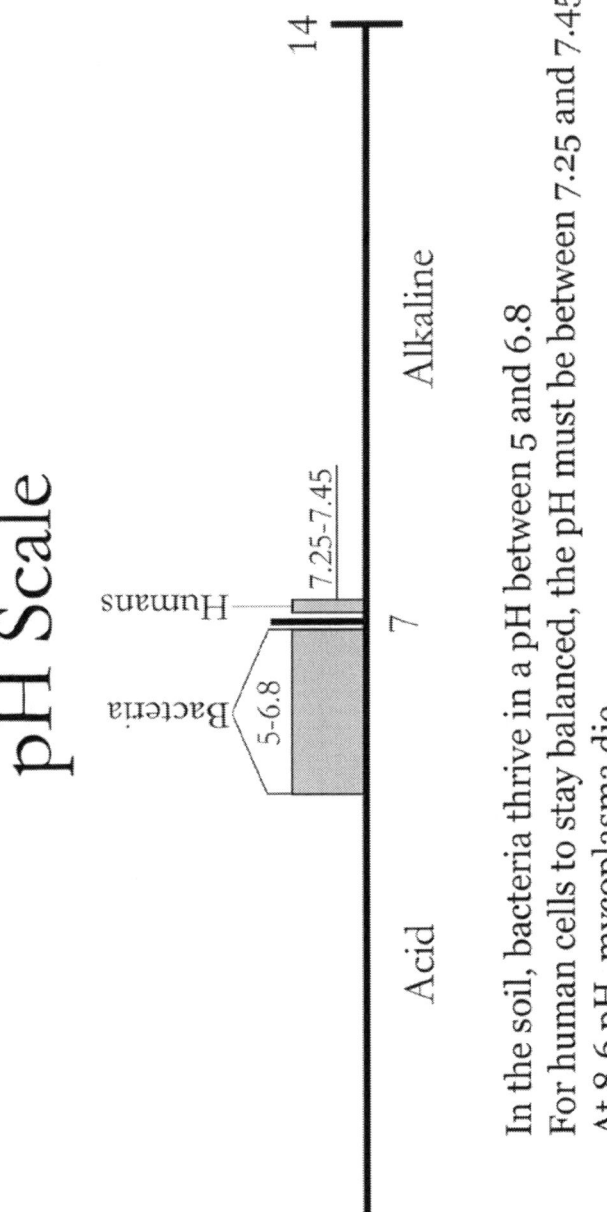

In the soil, bacteria thrive in a pH between 5 and 6.8
For human cells to stay balanced, the pH must be between 7.25 and 7.45
At 8.6 pH, mycoplasma die

It's No Acid-ent Why Some People Do Not Get Sick

Alkaline minerals are in fruits, vegetables, hazelnuts, Brazil nuts and almonds. Acidic minerals are phosphorous, sulfur, chlorine, iodine, bromine, manganese, fluorine, copper and silicon, to name a few, and found in meat, grains, nuts, soda, coffee, tea, preservatives, and processed foods.

When our cells burn molecules to make energy, not everything is burned. Minerals (consider them rock fragments) in the food we eat do not burn and are left as residual ash in the body's tissues and blood. Everyone has heard the phrase "You are what you eat!" This is true. The human body's pH is determined and measured by the mineral residue in the blood and tissues.

When the body is healthy and in perfect balance, its pH is alkaline, around 7.25 to 7.45, meaning there is a higher concentration of alkaline minerals in the blood and tissues than acid minerals.

Potential hydrogen (pH) is measured on a 0-14 scale. Any measurement below seven is acidic. Any measurement above seven is alkaline. Also, the closer the measurement is to zero, the greater the concentration of acidic minerals. On the other side of the scale, the closer the measurement is to 14, the greater the concentration of alkaline minerals. If the measurement is seven, the pH is neutral, neither acid nor alkaline.

Neutral means that the mineral concentration in the water has an equal amount of acidic minerals and alkaline minerals. It must also be noted that alkaline and acid minerals "bind" to each other (opposites attract), thus neutralizing each other. When this "binding" occurs, the pH becomes neutral, neither acid nor alkaline.

Just like the Universe (which must stay in perfect balance) so, too, must the human body's pH stay in perfect balance to remain healthy. There are several mechanisms in the body, which make this possible.

The first mechanism is referred to as the "great alkaline reserve," which keeps the blood's pH in perfect balance (alkaline). For every action, there is a reaction! When we eat too much food containing high concentrations of acid minerals, the body reacts by calling upon its "great alkaline reserve." Stored alkaline minerals are released into the bloodstream and "bind" to the acid minerals, thus neutralizing them. This causes the blood's pH to stabilize and return to perfect balance–an alkaline pH of ~7.25 to 7.45.

Too much acid mineral residue in the human tissues is toxic! To bring the body's tissues back to balance, there is another mechanism the body relies on–sweating. Our ancestors worked outside toiling in the hot sun, sweating out toxins through the skin. Unfortunately, this is not the case today. We live in air-conditioned houses, drive air-conditioned cars, and exercise in air-conditioned gymnasiums. We avoid sweating! Our ancestors also had an advantage over us. They did not have to contend with pollution, heavy metals, pesticides, herbicides, preservatives and many other chemicals, which are toxic to our cells. If these poisons are not sweated out, they remain in the cells and cause the cells to become "unbalanced." The cell's pH becomes acidic.

Besides using the above two mechanisms, the body has another way of ridding itself of too much acidic waste. It releases acid minerals through the kidneys and the colon. For our ancestors, this was ideal. Their diet consisted of large quantities of fruits, whole grains, vegetables, seeds, etc., which made elimination a quick process. However, today it's a different story. Most Americans' diets consist of large quantities of highly processed foods and meat, which contain a high concentration of acidic minerals and are very constipating. We also do not drink enough water. Thus, the elimination process is slowed down tremendously. When the elimination process slows down, the colon has a chance to reabsorb the toxins and put them right back into circulation, where they go right back into the tissues.

Finally, if the cells in our bodies are "unbalanced" (acid pH), this is when we become vulnerable to disease and cancer.

When we are told, "Eat your fruits and vegetables!" it's not just about getting our daily vitamin requirements. According to some experts, for the body to stay in perfect "balance," 80 percent of a person's diet must consist of food containing alkaline minerals and the remaining 20 percent consist of food containing acid minerals.

Why is there so much emphasis on this? Answer: It's because cancer and other disease-causing microorganisms (bacteria, fungus and viruses) cannot thrive in alkaline (balanced) tissues. In fact, bacteria (Lyme spirochaete is the exception) thrive in an acid environment of 5 to 6.8 (that is the ideal soil pH).

DID YOU KNOW?

Most bacteria remain dormant in an alkaline environment and die at a pH of 8.6!

VEGETABLES	Alkaline	Acid	VEGETABLES (cont'd)	Alkaline	Acid
Asparagus	H		Kale	M	
Beets	M		Kelp	EH	
Broccoli	M		Lettuce	M	
Brussels Sprouts	S		Leaf Lettuce	H	
Cabbage	M		Onions (depends on variety)	S-M	
Carrots	H		Parsley	EH	
Cauliflower	M		Peppers (Bell)	M	
Celery	H		Peppers (Cayenne)	EH	
Collard Greens	M		All Potatoes (with skin)	M	
Cucumbers	M		Pumpkin	M	
Eggplant	M		Spinach	H	
Endive/Escarole	H		Squash	M	
Garlic	H		Tomatoes (depends on variety)	S-M	

MINERAL CONCENTRATION

EH = Extremely high   H = High   M = Moderate   S = Slight

Ex: Tomatoes have a slight to moderate alkaline mineral concentration (a measurement somewhere between 7 and 10.5 on the pH scale).

```
        1.75   3.50   5.25        8.75  10.50  12.25
    |    |     |     |     |      |     |     |     |
  0 | EH |  H  |  M  |  S  |  S   |  M  |  H  | EH  | 14
         Acid              7           Alkaline
                        Neutral
```

FRUIT	Alkaline	Acid	FRUIT (cont'd)	Alkaline	Acid
Apples	M		Melons (all varieties)	EH	
Apricots	H		Mangos/Papayas	EH	
Avocados	H		Nectarines	H	
Bananas (ripe)	H		Oranges (with pulp)	M	
Blueberries		S	Peaches	M	
Cherries	M		Pears	H	
Cranberries		S	Pineapple	H	
Grapefruit	H		Plums/Prunes		S
Grapes	H		Raspberries	H	
Kiwi	H		Strawberries	H	
Lemons/Lines	EH		Tangerines	M	

MINERAL CONCENTRATION

EH = Extremely high   H = High   M = Moderate   S = Slight

Example: Honeydew and watermelon (all melons) have an extremely high concentration of alkaline minerals (a measurement somewhere between 12.25 and 14 on the pH scale).

```
        1.75   3.50   5.25        8.75  10.50  12.25
   |  EH  |  H  |  M  |  S  |  S  |  M  |  H  |  EH  |
   0         Acid         7         Alkaline         14
                       Neutral
```

68

MISCELLANEOUS	Alkaline	Acid	MISCELLANEOUS	Alkaline	Acid
Almonds (raw)	M		All processed meat		EH
All other nuts (raw)		S	Chicken/Beef		M
White Flour		H	Pork		H
Refined sugar		EH	Brown rice		M
Artificial sweetener		EH	White rice		H
Coffee		H	Beer/Liquor		H
Fast food		EH	Wine		M
Soda (regular & diet)		EH	Eggs (hard boiled)		M

MINERAL CONCENTRATION

EH = Extremely high   H = High   M = Moderate   S = Slight

Ex: Artificial sweeteners, fast food and soda contain an extremely high concentration of acid minerals.

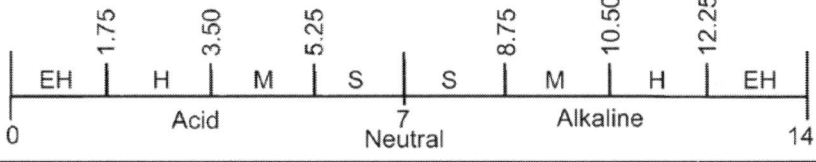

The Gerson Therapy

Today, Dr. Max Gerson, a German-born Jew who immigrated to the United States circa World War II, is considered to be the Father of Nutrition.

His theory was that cancer and disease are caused by: (1) a deficiency of nutrients and (2) toxins in the body.

Ostracized by allopathic medicine, he proved he was right by curing the incurable. He treated all types of cancer, some terminally ill, who had been told by their doctors they had months if not weeks to live.

In 1958, he published his first book, entitled, *A Cancer Therapy Results of 50 Cases*. Hundreds of thousands of copies were sold worldwide.

DID YOU KNOW?

When Dr. Gerson's first book was almost finished, he fell ill. After nursing himself back to health, he found that his manuscript had disappeared. Dr. Gerson then discovered that his secretary had been stealing his files and passing them on to another physician. He fired her and it took him another year to reconstruct another manuscript, published in 1958.

After publishing the rewritten manuscript, he fell ill again but this time the illness was fatal. Suspicious, before he died in 1959, he tested himself and confirmed that he had been poisoned with arsenic.

Had he died the first time he fell ill, his book would never have been published and the world would never have learned about and benefited from the Gerson Therapy.

Today, his daughter Charlotte has followed in her father's footsteps and has carried on his legacy, treating patients in a Tijuana Hospital.

Thousands from all over the world have journeyed to the Gerson Institute office located in San Diego, CA.

AUTHOR'S COMMENTS

A few of his patients were quite famous. He "cured" Dr. Albert Schweitzer of diabetes, along with Dr. Schweitzer's wife who had tuberculosis. He also treated their daughter for a skin disease--curing all of them by using the Gerson therapy.

In the movie The *Gerson Miracle*, his daughter Charlotte explains the treatment. She states that vegetables and fruits should be juiced to flood the body with nutrients and enzymes as fast as allowed. It is also noted that ALL vegetables and fruits used in the Gerson Therapy be organically grown, thus insuring their quality and effectiveness.

Dr. Gerson's cancer therapy (protocol) consisted of eating whole and juiced fresh and organic fruits and vegetables, along with supplements (including enzymes), and detoxing, the body (liver) with organic coffee enemas. In an astounding number of cases, cancer disappeared within a matter of weeks.

DID YOU KNOW?

It is against the law for an allopathic doctor to practice the Gerson Therapy in the United States.

Fat, Sick and Nearly Dead

This is a 2010 film, which follows Australian Joe Cross's 60-day journey across the United States. What makes this film so important is that it re-enforces "alkalizing the body" to kill pathogens.

As the title implies, Joe Cross was fat, sick and nearly dead. He was 41 years old, weighed 309 pounds and suffered from urticaria, an autoimmune disease (FYI: caused by mycoplasma).

In his journey across America, which started in New York City, he only drank what he referred to as "green juice."

After just 30 days of juicing, he lost 30 pounds. By day 61, he had lost 82 pounds. Eight weeks later, he was off his medication (steroids) and weighed 220. Not surprisingly, his urticaria symptoms disappeared.

On his journey, he interviewed many Americans about their eating habits and informed them about "rebooting" their systems.

The second half of the film is about a truck driver, Phil Staples, Joe Cross met in Arizona, who had the same autoimmune disease Joe had. Phil Staples, too, was tired of being fat, sick and nearly dead. He was 6'1", weighed 429 pounds and 42 years old.

In the documentary, Staples went on a 60-day juice fast and lost 91 pounds. Ten months later, Staples weighed 227, a total weight loss of 202 pounds! He also was able to get off all medications, which included methotrexate and steroids. Joe and Phil are now disease-free, meaning no mycoplasma infection.

AUTHOR'S COMMENTS

There were two factors, which reversed their autoimmune disease. One was they alkalized their bodies. The second, they stopped eating meat protein, explained in more detail in the Truth about Enzymes Chapter, page 194.

Baking Soda (NaHCO$_3$)

Sodium bicarbonate a/k/a baking soda is an alkaline chemical compound that has amazing cancer "cure" stories behind it. On a scale of 0 to 14 (seven being neutral), baking soda is 9, meaning it is super alkaline. (FYI: A pH of 8.6 kills mycoplasma.)

BENEFITS OF BAKING SODA

- Acidosis (helps alkalize body)
- Aspirin overdoses. (Aspirin requires an acidic environment for absorption and the alkaline properties [9] diminish aspirin absorption.)
- Relieves insect bites and stings (The topical formula is three parts baking soda to one part water.)
- Works as a cleanser of the teeth and gums, neutralizing the production of lactic acid (waste product of anaerobic bacteria) in the mouth
- Acts as an antiseptic to prevent infections (Most pathogens do not thrive in an alkaline environment.)
- Added to washing machines to eliminate odors
- Acts as a water softener
- Removes tea and coffee stains from cups
- Eliminates odors (place an open box of baking soda in the refrigerator)
- Used as a pesticide (Baking soda is registered by the EPA as a biopesticide.)

Mycoplasma can't survive for very long in a pH greater than 8, but this is dangerous for humans, too. Alkalosis occurs when the blood's pH exceeds 7.45. The perfect blood pH for humans is between 7.25 and 7.45. The perfect pH environment for bacteria is 5.0 to 6.8. (Alkalosis refers to the blood's pH and not to the cells' pH.)

DID YOU KNOW?

Baking soda can be used as toothpaste. BONUS: Any baking soda absorbed through the mouth helps alkalize the body!

The following story is about a man who fought stage IV prostate cancer (on his own) and won. He is becoming quite famous.

The Story of Vernon "Vito" Johnson

According to Vernon, in and around March of 2008, he visited a doctor and his PSA test results were 22+. In his story, he states the doctor then scheduled him for a biopsy.

The biopsy report indicated he had prostate cancer. Standard procedure was then followed for a bone scan because prostate cancer usually spreads (metastasizes) to the bones (pelvis).

DID YOU KNOW?

Bone is one of the most common locations for metastasis. For some reason, bone marrow tends to be the favorite metastases of breast cancer, prostate cancer and lung cancer. Further, normal healthy bone marrow produces <u>500</u> <u>billion</u> blood cells <u>a</u> <u>day</u>, plus it produces lymphocytes, which support the immune system. (Prostate cancer is caused by mycoplasmas.)

After the bone and pelvic scan results came in, the doctors diagnosed Vernon with aggressive prostate cancer and metastatic disease of the sacrum and pelvis.

FYI: Sacrum is the triangular bone at the base of the spine and at the upper and back part of the pelvic cavity. The pelvic cavity contains the reproductive organs, the urinary bladder, the colon, and the rectum.

Vernon then went to his primary care doctor for a second opinion and she sent him to an oncologist, who ran tests and confirmed the previous findings, except he found lesions within the pelvis, plus he added another diagnosis to the report--Stage IV cancer.

As he tells his story, Vernon's humor comes shining through when he writes about the oncologist's report, "What? Stage IV? Is that what I think it says? There is no Stage V!"

Vernon then goes on to say that the oncologist found spots that the first team of doctors had missed.

Vernon reflects how his son mentioned to him about pH and how pH affects the body. That is when Vernon started a quest--a search to find a treatment to kill the cancer.

(NOTE: Vernon was lucky. It sounds like the doctors had given up on him, because he did not mention being offered standard allopathic cancer [chemo] treatments.)

Vernon's research first led him to cesium chloride therapy, which he states "Eats up cancer. It attacks the tumor from the inside out."

Unfortunately, according to Vernon, his cesium order was lost in the mail, and that is when he found a backup plan--baking soda, which could also raise his body's pH.

He goes on to say that neither cesium nor baking soda research indicated it could help rid the body of bone cancer, but he decided to try anyway. He states that is when he decided to add Black Strap molasses as the "carrier."

He started his protocol on June 2, 2008 and quit the protocol on June 12, 2008, because he was scheduled for another bone scan on the 13th.

Miraculously, when he got this bone scan test results back, the report read, No convincing evidence of an osseous metastatic process. (FYI: meaning no sign of cancer)

Then a couple of days later, his PSA tests came back and they were 0.1. Vernon describes his experience as "Being Hit by a Rainbow."

AUTHOR'S COMMENTS

Vernon is different than the ordinary person who is diagnosed with stage IV cancer. He didn't give up by "buying" the doctors' diagnosis (death sentence). He chose to take charge of his destiny, took a chance and won.

He is now helping many people by telling his story and giving out his baking soda protocol on his web site. Congratulations Vernon! You are an inspiration.

www.phkillscancer.com

The Story of Dr. Simoncini

Dr. Simoncini, an Italian doctor, prescribes the same protocol used by Vernon, but he also intravenously injects baking soda solution directly into the tumor or infected area. For his oral protocol visit:

www.cancertutor.com/Cancer02/Simoncini.html

He also developed a protocol that intravenously injects the baking soda into the cancer site. Visit Dr. Simoncini's official web site:

www.cancerfungus.com

His story began when he questioned a professor in medical school as to the cause of cancer. The professor's answer was that they didn't know. This conversation sparked his questioning allopathic medicine.

Dr. Simoncini stands apart from allopathic medical practitioners. He states his theory in the title of his book, *Cancer is a Fungus*. As an oncologist, he noticed that "fungus" was present in cancerous tumors. He also states that especially Candida is present in cancer. In his book, he questions useless studies and experimentation with poisons:

> ".......so that nobody understands anything while the scientific impotence and the inadequacies of the current oncological systems are kept in the dark."

According to Dr. Simoncini, the average cancer patient's treatments costs well over $300,000 and that the published survival rate of cancer patients is false--that it is too high.

DID YOU KNOW?

Dr. Simoncine's license to practice was taken away from him in Italy, but he has many followers who steadfastly believe in his protocol.

He is featured in the documentary movie, *Cancer: The Forbidden Cures*.

Baking Soda and Lemon Juice Protocol

You will need:

1. Two ounces of fresh lemon Juice

2. One-half teaspoon aluminum-free baking soda (Arm & Hammer or Bob's)

STEP 1

Put baking soda and lemon juice in a glass. Add six to eight ounces of purified water.

DOSAGE

Twice a day

7 Lemons a Day Keep the Mycoplasma Away

According to R Webster Kehr of www.cancertutor.com, this protocol is not alkalizing enough to interfere with the baking soda protocol.

STEP 1

Freeze six lemons each day (including skin).

Cut off stem of each lemon before freezing.

After freezing, grate and eat two lemons three times per day.

Author's Comments

Watch this protocol on youTube.

Baking Soda and Maple Syrup Protocol

The principle behind this protocol is to get the baking soda inside the cancer cell to kill the mycoplasmas. Mycoplasmas need sugar and the maple syrup/molasses/honey is a "carrier."

For this protocol to be effective, consume absolutely NO meat, dairy, sugar, or white flour during this protocol. The theory is the mycoplasmas need sugar and will feed only on the baking soda/sugar mixture. The baking soda will raise the cell's pH and the mycoplasmas will die.

According to sources, this is a highly alkalizing protocol. Do this protocol no longer than six weeks.

The ratio is one teaspoon of baking soda to three teaspoons of (your choice) maple syrup, molasses or honey.

Make multiple dosages and store at room temperature.

STEP 1

In a non-aluminum saucepan, add the correct ratio (1 teaspoon of baking soda to 3 teaspoons of maple syrup, molasses or honey).

STEP 2

Heat mixture on very low heat, stirring until baking soda dissolves. (If mixture tastes bad, you have burned it.)

STEP 3

Take one teaspoon of mixture four times a day, which is the equivalent of one teaspoon of baking soda a day.

WARNING: According to sources, an advanced cancer patient can take up to 16 teaspoons of mixture per day, but this should only be for a maximum of one week! (Sixteen teaspoons of mixture per day equals four teaspoons of baking soda per day.)

Calcium Protocol

Alkalizing the Body

For calcium to be absorbed properly by the body, D3 must be present. Also supplementing with Vitamin C through fruits and vegetables is crucial for absorption.

The following calcium protocol gradually alkalizes your body to avoid Heerxheimer's reaction (immune system response to die-off) and is from cancertutor.com:

Week One

One pill three times a day at mealtime

Week Two through Six

Two pills three times a day at mealtime.

Week Seven

One pill three times a day and thereafter.

Author's Comments

R. Webster Kehr of cancertutor.com warns that if you take a multivitamin, and if it includes Vitamin D3, do not take additional dosage of D3.

The calcium should be 100 percent pure coral calcium.

Visit Webster's web site for other effective cancer protocols:

www.cancertutor.com

Section 3

"Detoxing" the Cells

Sulfur (Detox)

Not only is sulfur used to treat cancer and disease, but it is also an essential element for all life. Sulfur deficiency will lead to cell degeneration then on to disease or cancer.

Sulfur deficiency can be a factor in joint pain, back pain, sore muscles, headaches, heartburn, cold sores, gray hair, gastrointestinal disorders, acne, just to name a few.

Sulfur plays a key role in oxygenation (oxygen transporter) and detoxification of the cells. There is a correlation between sulfur deficiency and chlorine/fluoride intake, both of which inhibit sulfur absorption in the body.

Sulfur has other important roles in the body:

- Is largely responsible for the mechanical strength and insolubility of the protein keratin found in the skin and hair
- Disulfide bonds are a major component in holding joints and connective tissue together, making cartilage firm and resilient

It is vital to ingest an organic (not a by-product) form of sulfur. It is also important to buy plant-derived sulfur in a crystalline state. Powdered (capsules) sulfur is not a choice.

WARNING: Sulfur thins blood. It can also enhance prescriptions. To be safe, before taking sulfur supplements, consult your doctor.

DID YOU KNOW?

China is one of the main suppliers of sulfur supplements, which are contaminated by-products of natural gas and petroleum. Just because the packaging may say "manufactured in America" does not guarantee the sulfur did not come from China.

Many people are allergic to sulfur. I suspect they are allergic to the powdered Chinese sulfur that is a by-product of natural gas. Usually when I question someone who is allergic to sulfur, I find out he or she is not allergic to cruciferous vegetables. I am sure there are other reputable sulfur vendors, but I trust and buy my organic sulfur from the following vendor:

http://www.h20airwateramericas.com

Tony Isaac's Liver Cleanse Protocol

Dr. Max Gerson observed cancer could not develop unless the liver was impaired.

When you kill pathogens, the pathogens (mycoplasma) release endotoxins, which heavily tax the liver. The release of these toxins can overwhelm an already weakened liver and cause the immune system to respond (Herxheimer). The following liver cleanse can help regenerate the liver:

Five Day Liver Cleanse

NOTE: It is suggested that day four be on a Saturday or at a time when you can stay home.

Day 1: Drink one liter (four cups) of apple juice during the day. Eat normally.

Day 2: Drink another liter of apple juice. Eat normally.

Day 3: Drink another liter of apple juice. Eat normally.

Day 4: Do not eat any solid food after lunchtime. At 6 pm take one level tablespoon of Epsom salt in a glass of water. At 8 pm take another tablespoon of Epsom salt in a glass of water. At 10 pm mix one-half glass of olive oil and three-quarter glass of freshly squeezed grapefruit juice. Pour into a jar with a lid and shake well. Drink mixture and get into bed after drinking the mixture.

Day 5: You may be taking more than one trip to the toilet during the night of Day 4, as well as during Day 5.

FYI: Tony Isaac is famous for his oleander soup protocol.

Ion Footbath (Detox and Alkalize)

The following is a seller's description of the ionic footbath:

> "The ion foot bath is a holistic way of approaching disease through saturation of the blood, tissues, cells and organs with ions. These treatments are based on ionization of water and osmosis to draw toxins from the body. The ion foot bath produces negative hydrogen ions in the water and ions act as both an energy carrier and as an antioxidant in the human body."

Many users claim it:

- Enhances body detoxification and helps lose weight
- Inactivates viruses, bacteria, yeast, and fungus
- Reduces pain and inflammation and relieves tension
- Slows down many conditions associated with old age
- Purifies blood and lymph and chelates heavy metals
- Increases energy
- Stimulates the immune system"

Ion footbaths range from very expensive to moderately reasonable. If you are interested in buying an ion foot detox, check out this web site:

www.ionspa.com

The Story of Dr. Hazel Parcells

Dr. Hazel Parcells was an instructor in the 1950s at Sierra States University in Los Angeles. Her focus was on nutrition, detoxification and energy healing. She discovered when electro-magnetic fields are blocked from shock and/or trauma, toxins are held in cells and are not released. She developed techniques that corrected these energy field blockages.

Another important discovery she made is what made her famous worldwide. During the 1950s, while conducting research in nutrition and food preparation, she was experimenting with old lemons. When she soaked these lemons in a sink filled with water and a small amount of Clorox bleach, she noticed that the fruit rejuvenated--in appearance and odor. She then cut up the "refreshed" lemons and froze them. Over the next three years, she tested these same lemons and discovered that they had the same nutrition and freshness as "fresh" lemons. This discovery became known as "The Parcells Oxygen Soak."

Sodium Hypochlorite (NaClO)

Sodium hypoclorite works as an oxygenator in Clorox and as a disinfectant. It eliminates the breakdown of food by destroying fungus and bacteria. Clorox also removes pesticides, toxins and other chemicals from food, extending fruit and vegetable life. (FYI: Clorox is not the same as chlorine used to purify drinking water. Sodium hypochlorite breaks down into salt and water.)

Chemical Reaction

When Clorox is added to water, a chemical reaction occurs. Electrons, freed by the dilution of Clorox, cause the sodium hypochlorite to "clean" fruits and vegetables, killing fungus and bacteria. The release of strong <u>negative</u> ions pulls <u>positively</u> charged ions (toxins and pesticides) out of the produce. (Remember? Opposites attract)

Dr. Parcells found that Clorox was the best, theorizing that the company's filtration systems and use of stainless steel made their product superior to others. For more information about Dr. Parcells and parasite/toxin cleansing protocols visit:

www.parcellscenter.com

Dr. Parcells lived to be 106. Dr. Parcells' protocol for soaking food is next.

The Parcells Oxygen Soak

Step One

Add one teaspoon of Clorox bleach to one gallon of water. Do not mix different types of vegetables and fruits together. Each type requires different soak times.

Type of Food	Minutes
Leafy vegetables (lettuces)	5-10
Root Vegetables (beets, potatoes, radishes, etc.)	10-15
Fruits (thin-skinned) [ex: berries]	5
Fruits (medium skinned) [ex: peaches, plums, grapes]	10
Fruits (thick-skinned) [apples, citrus]	10-15
Eggs (in shell)	20-30
Meats (per pound)	10
Meats (frozen, per pound)	15-20

Step Two

After soaking vegetables/fruits/meats for recommended time, rinse them in fresh water, which will clean off any chemicals and reintroduce oxygen to the food.

Step Three

Shake lettuce and drain all soaked food before refrigerating.

Author's Comments

This soak should eliminate the need to buy expensive organic foods. This soak will remove pesticides and toxins and prolong shelf life of your food.

Section 4

"Protecting" Yourself from Cancer and Disease

The Ketogenic Diet

America is under siege. One hundred percent of the population is infected with mycoplasma, even if they do not show symptoms yet. It is impossible not to be infected, unless a person has lived in a sterile environment from birth and was delivered Caesarean. (Once the mycoplasma has been transmitted, mycoplasmas lie dormant in degenerative cells—even in children, waiting for an opportunity to awaken.)

Protect yourself from cancer or disease (especially mycoplasma), adopt a ketogenic diet, even it is a modified ketogenic diet. This diet absolutely avoids the standard American diet, which is high in sugar. Fat intake represents 75-80% of the diet. (FYI: Fat turns into ketones, which are fuel for the brain and body.)

The logic behind this diet is that mycoplasma metabolizes sugar; and without sugar, it starves and will die.

The diet does allow carbohydrate intake, but only 5-10% of the total calories consists of "good" carbs.

Meat is allowed, but too much meat intake causes meat to turn into glucose, which defeats the purpose of the diet. Only 10-15% of the diet is from protein.

The following is a list of "good" carbohydrates:

VEGETABLES AND FRUIT (5-10% of calories)

Arugala, artichokes, asparagus, bok choy, broccoli, Brussels sprouts cabbage, cauliflower, celery, cucumbers, eggplant, garlic, green beans, jicama, kale, leeks, lettuce, mushrooms, okra, onions, parsley, peppers, pumpkin, radishes, radicchio, rhubarb, scallions, shallots, snow peas, spaghetti squash, summer squash, tomatoes, water cress, wax beans and zucchini

ALLOWABLE FRUIT (5-10% of calories)

Blackberries, blueberries, cranberries, lemons, limes, raspberries and strawberries

PROTEIN (10-15% of calories)

Bacon, beef, beef jerky, beef roast, bratwurst, chicken (skin on), duck, eggs (whole), fish, ground beef, goose, ham, hot dogs, kielbasa, pepperoni, pheasant, pork chops, pork ribs, pork rinds, pork roast, quail, salami, sausages, shellfish, steak, tuna, turkey and veal

FATS (75-80% of calories)

Almonds, almond butter, almond oil, avocado, avocado oil, bee_ blue cheese, Brazil nuts, butter, cheese, chia seeds, chicken fat, coconut, coconut cream, coconut milk (unsweetened), coconut oil, cream cheese, dark chocolate (75% cacao), fish oil, flaxseed and oil, ghee, Greek yogurt (plain and low sugar), heavy whipping cream, hemp seed and oil, lard, Macadamia nuts, mayonnaise, olive oil (extra virgin), pecans, pistachios, sour cream, sunflower seeds and walnuts

AUTHOR'S COMMENTS

Absolutely no citrus fruit, juices, bananas, apples, grapes, etc., are allowed under fruit--just those on the list.

Notice there are no potatoes, carrots, grains, or beans allowed.

Absolutely no alcohol or soda is allowed.

For a sweetener, use stevia.

For more information, there are web sites dedicated to the ketogenic diet.

AUTHOR'S COMMENTS

This diet is a <u>must</u> for someone who has an "active" mycoplasma infection, including cancer. If you are not sick (yet), this lifestyle diet will help protect you from mycoplasma.

Bovine Colostrum

Female mammals' breasts produce colostrum after birthing, which is very important for the survival of the newborn. Cows are the universal donors of colostrum. Colostrum is rich in:

- Enzymes
- Amino acids, vitamin A and sodium
- IGF-1 (insulin-like growth factor one)
- Medium-chain fatty acids
- Antibodies
- Immune cells (T cells)
- Antibodies (IgA, IgC, and IgM)
- Lactoferin

IGF-1

IGF-1 is a hormone that is similar in structure to insulin. It is important for growth in young children. It contains 70 amino acids in a single chain.

IGF-1 is produced throughout life and the highest output is during puberty. The lowest levels of output are during infancy and old age.

Newborns have a very immature digestive system and IGF-1 is readily absorbed (not digested) into the bloodstream. However, since IGF-1 is a protein, in adults, it is rapidly broken down in the gastrointestinal tract.

On a positive note, when the pituitary gland manufactures growth hormones (GH), GH is released into the bloodstream and stimulates the liver to produce IGF-1.

A few benefits of IGF-1 include:

- Skeletal system development
- DNA replication
- Muscle/organ development

AUTHOR'S COMMENTS

To benefit from IGF-1, colostrum could be absorbed through the mucus membranes in the mouth to avoid destructive digestion.

T Cells

T cells (lymphocytes) are manufactured in the thymus gland, which is a major component of the immune system. Each T cell attacks a specific pathogen that it has identified in the past. The mother's T cells are passed on to its newborn in colostrum. Thus, any pathogen the mother has encountered, the newborn's immune system will attack that particular pathogen.

According to Wikipedia:

> "Bovine colostrum from pasture-fed cows contains immunoglobulins specific to many human pathogens, including E. coli, Cryptosporidium parvum, Shigella flexneri, Salmonella, Staphylococcus and rotavirus"

FACT: Before the introduction of vaccines, colostrum was the main source of immunoglobulins used to fight infections. Dr. Albert Sabin used colostrum immunoglobulins in his first oral vaccine against polio.

DID YOU KNOW?

At birth, the thymus gland is the size of a small navel orange. By the age of 25, the thymus begins to atrophy and is slowly replaced by fat. By the age of 70, the size of the thymus is one-third of what it was at birth.

According to Wikipedia:

> "The stock of T-lymphocytes is built up in early life, so the function of the thymus is diminished in adults. It is largely degenerated in elderly adults and is barely identifiable, consisting mostly of fatty tissue, but it continues its endocrine function." (Note: Endocrine refers to hormones.)

Lactoferin

Lactoferin is a multifunctional protein and is a component of the immune system. Its main function is transporting iron ions to cells and controlling the level of free iron in the blood. It has antibacterial, antiviral and anti-parasitic functions and properties, too.

Bacteria and other microorganisms need iron. Lactoferin sequesters free roaming iron in the bloodstream, thus blocking bacterial growth. According to Wikipedia:

> "Lactoferin binds to lipopolysaccharides in bacterial walls and the oxidized iron part of the lactoferin oxidizes bacteria via

formation of peroxides. This affects the membrane permeability and results in the cell breakdown."

NOTE: Amazingly, Wikipedia is describing the mycoplasma endotoxin, a lipopolysaccharide.

There is more. Lactoferin also:

- Stimulates phagocytosis (immune response)
- Disrupts the membrane and penetrates into the cell wall of the bacterium
- Inhibits (prevents) the attachment of H. pylori in the stomach, hence preventing ulcers
- Prevents the formation of bacterial biofilm (plaque)

Lactoferin has anti-viral functions. It binds to cell membranes, which repels viruses. (Viruses bind to lipoproteins of the cell membranes and then penetrate the cell.)

Researchers have discovered that lactoferin levels in tear fluid (eyes) decreases dry eye diseases such as Sjogren's syndrome. (This is caused by mycoplasma.)

Another study discovered increased formation of biofilm due to decreased levels of lactoferin was observed in patients with cystic fibrosis.

Colostrum has a mild laxative effect on the newborn, which stimulates the baby's first stool.

According to Wikipedia:

> "There is a purpose to this laxative effect. It clears out waste products of dead red blood cells, which are produced at birth due to blood volume reduction from the baby's body. Colostrum also helps prevent jaundice."

Athletes and body builders use colostrum to enhance muscles and speed up muscle healing. Colostrum also helps in the healing process after surgeries. (I can vouch for that.)

Sellers of bovine colostrum suggest taking colostrum supplements on an empty stomach to keep it from going through the digestive process.

Colostrum is available at health food stores, Amazon, or other sites on the Internet.

The Story of AZOMITE

Rollin J. Anderson was a geological prospector from San Francisco, California, who started a mining company in 1942 to mine and sell a "pink" ore discovered in central Utah. He had heard about the Native American Indian folklore regarding the healing powers of the "painted rock" just south of Salt Lake City.

He took a sample of the "pink" rock to a friend, Charles Head, who was a microscopist at the U.S. Bureau of Mines. The analysis showed an array of minerals similar to "caliche" rock only found in Chili and Peru. (Experts believe that this "caliche" rock represents most of the world's source for nitrate. See definitions for caliche and nitrate at the end of this chapter.)

The "painted rock" contained over 70 trace minerals, which prompted Anderson to name his discovery AZOMITE, which is an acronym for A to Z Of Minerals Including Trace Elements = AZOMITE (all caps).

According to Wikipedia:

> "AZOMITE is a registered trademark for a complex silica ore unique to the Utah mineral deposit from which it is mined. When the ash from a volcanic eruption filled a nearby seabed an estimated 30 million years ago, the combination of seawater fed by hundreds of mineral rich rivers and the rare earth minerals in the volcanic ash created the deposit's distinctive composition."

Anderson believed that benefits derived from nitrates were actually from trace elements, which served as catalysts.

He first proved his theory with tomatoes. AZOMITE added to the soil yielded healthier and stronger tomatoes, free from worm infestation. It also helped plants better absorb nutrients from the soil.

He then tried AZOMITE on livestock and got amazing results:

- Greater egg production with less breakage
- Improvement in growth, reproductive vigor and immunity
- Better absorption of feed = less cost to farmers
- Increased milk production

According to Wikipedia:

"Agriculture and livestock producers have used AZOMITE to support livestock health and plant nutrition for over 70 years."

Currently approved for livestock consumption, AZOMITE is also approved for agriculture. Of course, the FDA has not approved AZOMITE for human consumption.

DID YOU KNOW?

Thirty percent of AZOMITE is sold internationally in over 30 countries.

When Anderson retired in 1988, he leased the reserves to the mining company Peak Minerals. In 2011, the Anderson Company merged with another company and became Azomite Mineral Products, Inc.

Author's Comments

Nutritional experts describe AZOMITE as a "super food." Organic gardeners use it to enhance their soil. AZOMITE contains all the essential minerals and trace minerals in a balanced ratio. The company grinds up the rock small enough that it can pass through cell walls.

Lastly, AZOMITE is "dirt cheap."

Definitions

<u>Caliche</u> - A sedimentary rock made up of *calcium carbonate. Used to build structures, Caliche binds materials such as gravel, sand, clay and silt. FYI: Caliche is Spanish for "lime."

> *Calcium carbonate is a chemical compound ($CaCO_3$) and is the main component of marine organism shells, snails, pearls and eggshells.

<u>Nitrate</u> (NO_3^-) - A source of nitrates in the human body comes from leafy green foods such as spinach. According to Wikipedia:

> "It is now believed that dietary nitrate in the form of plant-based foods is converted to nitrite. Nitrite and water are converted to nitric oxide (NO), which reduces hypertension."

Diatomaceous Earth

Diatomaceous earth (DE) is sedimentary rock consisting of fossilized remains of diatoms (hard-shelled single-celled algae). According to sources, diatomaceous earth dates back to the Jurassic period.

DE consists of 80+ percent silica, which is a very important element in the human body.

DE was first discovered by Peter Kasten, a peasant who was sinking a well on the slopes of north Germany. Today, diatomaceous earth is also mined in Nevada, Oregon, Washington, and California.

DID YOU KNOW?

Alfred Nobel used diatomaceous earth in the manufacturing of dynamite.

According to Wikipedia:

> "In 1860, Alfred Nobel discovered that nitroglycerin could be made much more stable if absorbed in diatomite. This allows much safer transport and handling than nitroglycerin in its raw form. He patented this mixture as dynamite in 1867."

On a hardness scale of one to ten, diamonds are a nine and DE is a seven. Its many benefits are:

A NATURAL PESTICIDE

Used in the storage of grains to combat insect infestation, diatomaceous earth, upon contact, absorbs moisture from an insect's' exoskeleton. This causes the bug's death due to dehydration.

NOTE: An insect's exoskeleton is composed of chitin. Chitin is a derivative of glucose and is the main component of cell walls of fungi (mold, yeast and mushrooms) and the exoskeletons of crustaceans (crabs, lobsters and shrimp).

ANTI-FUNGAL

Silica is absorbent. In the bloodstream, silica meets up with parasites, i.e., yeast and mold and absorbs the moisture from the parasite's cell wall (chitin). This then causes the parasite's death.

ANTI-BACTERIAL

Silica absorbs lipids, which is one of the components of mycoplasma membrane (lipopolysaccharide), causing the death of the mycoplasma.

ANTI-PARASITE (PETS AND PEOPLE)

Diatomaceous earth dries out and cuts the exoskeleton of tapeworms. (Sources report that it may take a month to kill the worms and eggs.)

LOWERS CHOLESTEROL

According to many sources, after taking DE, users have experienced LDL levels dropping. NOTE: DE absorbs LDL (low-density lipoprotein) and many people state their "bad" cholesterol dropped 40-50 points.

BLOOD PRESSURE

There are many testimonials that DE lowered their blood pressure. (NOTE: A possible explanation could be that because DE is "gritty", scouring the blood vessels and colon and scraping off the plaque.)

CAT LITTER

Non-food grade diatomaceous earth forms the "clumps" in cat litter.

TOOTHPASTE

The grit in toothpaste is diatomaceous earth.

MINERAL AND VITAMIN ABSORBTION

Bones cannot absorb calcium without silica. Silica is responsible for the depositing of minerals into the bones, especially calcium.

Silica speeds up the healing process of fractures and reduces scarring at the site of the fracture. Research has proven that when calcium is insufficient, the body will turn silica into calcium the body needs.

HAIR AND SKIN CARE

Silica is a main component of hair. Silica stimulates hair growth and is responsible for its strength.

Collagen is mostly made of silica, and collagen is the "glue" that holds us together. If the body has enough silica glucosaminoglycane, the collagen will make us look younger. Collagen enhances the skin elasticity. Collagen is also the main component of connective tissue and bone.

DETOX

DE (in the gut) detoxes heavy metals (aluminum and mercury), excreting the toxins and metals through the urinary tract.

TEETH AND GUMS

By hardening the enamel, silica prevents cavities and gum atrophy.

NAILS

DE strengthens the fingernails, making them less prone to break.

AUTHOR'S COMMENTS

Diatomaceous earth does sound too good to be true but seeing is believing. In my case, I started taking diatomaceous earth and within six months I no longer had to take pain medication because of joint pain. Further, from chronic rheumatoid arthritis, my left knee was in very bad shape. I feared knee replacement because my right knee had already been replaced. Amazingly, after ingesting DE for six months, my left knee has healed.

BEWARE: Use food grade diatomaceous earth. Crystalline diatomaceous earth used in swimming pool filters is harmful if breathed into the lungs. Swimming pool DE is also chemically treated and is, therefore, deadly if ingested.

SUMMARY (Some Benefits of DE)

- Cleanses colon naturally
- Enhances bowel movements
- Smooth and healthy skin
- Lowers bad cholesterol
- Fades age spots
- Repairs joints and ligaments
- Stronger teeth, nails and gums
- Natural pesticide, anti-microbial and anti-fungal

Sources recommend one teaspoon of diatomaceous earth in a glass of water or juice to test tolerance and then slowly building up the dosage. I love diatomaceous earth and I believe in it wholeheartedly. I put a heaping one-fourth cup of DE in my smoothie every morning.

To benefit from diatomaceous earth in the reconstruction of bones and collagen, you must have adequate amounts of Vitamin C. If Vitamin C is not present, your body cannot heal. People with chronic mycoplasma infections (cancer and disease) are deficient in Vitamin C, other vitamins and minerals.

WARNING

Diatomaceous earth acts as a clotting agent in the blood. People who are on blood thinners should not take diatomaceous earth unless approved by a doctor. Diatomaceous earth is super absorbent. Drink plenty of water to prevent dehydration.

Section 5

"Defending" Yourself with Plant-Based Phytochemicals

Introduction

> Let your food be your medicine and your medicine be your food — Hippocrates

Plants have evolved over time and produce defensive chemical compounds. These compounds are referred to as anti-herbivory. Officially (Wikipedia), there are three groups of anti-herbivory compounds:

- **Nitrogen-based**
- Terpenes (referred to as terpenoids)
- Phenols (includes flavonoids)

The focus of this "Defending" Yourself with Plant-Based Phytochemicals Section is **nitrogen** and **nitrogen/sulfur**-based chemical compounds, which are anti-microbial/anti-cancer. (Nitrogen and sulfur kill microorganisms and insects.) These are plants' natural defensive mechanisms.

There are three subgroups in the **nitrogen-based** chemical compound group. They are:

1. Alkaloids - Some of these nitrogen-based chemical compounds are nicotine, caffeine, morphine, strychnine and quinine. FYI: Nitrogen-based phytochemicals end in "ine," but this does not mean ALL phytochemicals ending in "ine" are alkaloids.

2. Glucosinolates - This **nitrogen**-based subgroup has a **sulfur** element attached. Examples of plants high in glucosinolates are broccoli, Brussels sprouts, and cabbage.

3. Cyanogenic Glycosides - These chemical compounds have a **cyanide** group in the formula, such as Amygdalin, which is present in certain grasses, apricot seeds, apple seeds, cherry seeds, plum seeds, crabapple seeds, peach seeds, etc.

1. Alkaloids

Alkaloids affect <u>cell</u> <u>membrane</u> (ex: mycoplasma endotoxin) and cytoskeletal (the cell's "skeleton," which is located inside the cell and is made of protein) structure causing the cells to weaken, collapse, and affect nerve transmission. Plant families usually have alkaloids in common. The following are families and plants that contain alkaloids. The following are good for protection, but they do not contain the "potent" alkaloids, that kill bacteria, fungus and viruses. Plants that contain potent alkaloids deserve their own chapters. (NOTE: Alkaloids taste "bitter".)

THE NIGHTSHADE FAMILY

<u>CHILI PEPPERS</u> are known for their "red hot" alkaloid Capsaicin.

<u>EGGPLANT</u> In this family, it contains the second highest concentration of nicotine, right behind tobacco. It has at least six alkaloids in the skin.

<u>POTATOES</u> are nonpoisonous if eaten in moderation. The skin contains at least ten alkaloids. One of the common alkaloids in the Nightshade family is nicotine. Nicotine is present in very low levels in fresh potatoes. Cooking or frying potatoes reduces the alkaloid content by 40-50%. Potato "eyes" and shoots contain high concentrations of alkaloids. For safety, avoid eating the eyes (buds), shoots or green potatoes.

<u>TOMATOES</u> are nonpoisonous if eaten in moderation. The skin contains at least ten alkaloids. Nicotine is present in very low levels in fresh tomatoes. WARNING: Avoid eating any part of the tomato plant, stems, leaves and raw green tomatoes. The alkaloids in the tomato plant are deadly to dogs, too.

FYI: Like potatoes, frying green tomatoes reduces the alkaloid content by 40-50%.

<u>WOLFBERRIES</u> are a very important industry in China and used medicinally by the Chinese for thousands of years. The alkaloid atropine is in Wolfberries. Atropine can cross the blood-brain barrier.

BETALAINS (Type of Alkaloid)

Betalains are classified as alkaloids and are present in beets, Swiss chard, pursalane and prickly pear cactus. According to studies, betalains have fungicidal properties.

BEETS Scientific studies found that drinking beet juice lowers blood pressure and proved that nitrates (betalain) open up the blood vessels and increase blood flow. Beets contain at least eight alkaloids.

PRICKLY PEAR CACTUS has a wide range of alkaloids.

PURSLANE is amazing, nutritious, non-toxic and a common backyard weed. It resembles a small version of a jade plant. It has green succulent leaves and grows well in any condition of soil. It contains alkaloids. Plant it in your garden!

SPINACH is very rich in nitrogen-based phytochemicals, which gives it its dark green color. Besides being nutritious, it is anti-microbial.

SWISS CHARD Swiss chard's leaves are green, but the stalks can vary (usually red). Swiss chard is in the same family as spinach, beets, and quinoa. One of its alkaloids is a powerful anti-oxidant, and studies have shown it has anti-cancer and anti-microbial properties.

OTHER PLANTS (in alphabetical order)

BLACK PEPPER has at least eight alkaloids.

CACAO (Chocolate) contains the alkaloid theobromine, which is very bitter. Dark chocolate has 2 to 2-1/2 times theobromine than milk chocolate. According to Wikipedia, the first Europeans to discover the cacao bean were Christopher Columbus and his crew. FYI: A cacao tree takes 4-5 years to reach maturity when it can start bearing fruit.

CARROT roots are very high in nitrogen/alkaloids. There are documented cases of cancer patients getting well by drinking only fresh carrot juice. Carrots used for juicing should be organic as carrots absorb toxins from the ground. The bitterness in the root means the presence of nitrogen/alkaloids. Don't peal carrots!

COFFEE has several alkaloids (caffeine), which are natural pesticides. The seeds (beans) of the coffee plant contain caffeine, which is a natural pesticide that paralyzes and kills certain insects feeding on the plant.

CUCUMBERS Think green. Green means the presence of nitrogen. Cucumber peel is high in nitrogen.

FENUGREEK is cultivated worldwide and is a common ingredient in Indian (India) dishes. Several studies have shown that it has an anti-diabetic effect on patients with type II diabetes.

LICORICE ROOT is used in traditional Chinese medicine. It is also in the Hoxsey anti-cancer formula, which is in a forthcoming chapter. Licorice root and fenugreek are in the same family.

POPPY SEED This plant has the most documented alkaloids in the entire plant kingdom. Twenty-five percent of the Opium Poppy's molecular structure is alkaloids. According to sources, morphine is in all parts of the plant, including the seeds.

Plants that have powerful medicinal alkaloids are listed under Section 6 – "Killing." Pathogens.

2. Glucosinolates

Glucosinolates contain <u>both</u> sulfur and nitrogen (CHNOS). Some of the vegetables in the Cruciferous family containing glucosinolates are: Horseradish, Horseradish Tree (Moringa), kale, collard greens, cabbage, Brussels sprouts, broccoflower, broccoli, cauliflower, Chinese cabbage, turnips, rutabaga, mustard seeds, watercress, radish, and bok choy.

FYI: Glucosinolates help rid the body of cancer-causing toxins. Glucosinolates activate the liver to produce enzymes that break down carcinogens to a harmless inactive form.

THE CRUCIFEROUS FAMILY

These vegetables can interfere with prescription drugs. According to Wikipedia, they can also cause goiters, since their enzymes interfere with the formation of the thyroid hormone in people with an iodine deficiency.

<u>BROCCOLI</u> This vegetable closely resembles cauliflower. It has many glucosinolate–nine. FYI: Microwaving or boiling broccoli in water will diminish its anti-microbial effectiveness. Boiling water leaches the nutrients and microwaving destroys the enzymes. Stir frying and steaming are the best.

<u>BRUSSELS SPROUTS</u> This vegetable has at least four glucosinoates.

<u>CABBAGE</u> This vegetable has at least 26 glucosinolates and at least one alkaloid. Cabbage is good for the eyes. It contains Lutein and Zeaxanthin.

<u>CAULIFLOWER</u> has at least 17 glucosinoates. FYI: Never boil cauliflower, as the enzymes will be destroyed and the glucosinolates will leach into the water. The ideal method is steaming, which does not diminish the potency of the alkaloids and glucosinolates. A study showed that a high intake of cauliflower reduced prostate cancer risk.

<u>HORSERADISH</u> This vegetable has more glucosinolates than broccoli–13!

<u>KALE</u> The only difference between kale and cabbage is that kale does not form a "head." Kale contains several glucosinolates. Kale contains both lutein and zeaxanthin. FYI: Kale freezes well, tastes sweeter and is more flavorful after being exposed to frost. When baked or dehydrated, kale takes on the consistency similar to that of a potato chip.

MORINGA Known as the Horseradish tree, studies show eating moringa can: be anti-aging; be anti-ulcer; be anti-cancer; be anti-tumor; be anti-inflammatory; and lowers cholesterol. Moringa has a high concentration of sulfur in its "dried" leaves—more than when the leaves were green. Did you know the leaves of the moringa contain: seven times the vitamin C of an organge, four times the calcium of milk, four times the potassium in a banana, and five times the vitamin A in carrots?

MUSTARD SEED At least nine glucosinolates are in mustard seeds, plus at least one alkaloid. FYI: Black mustard is in Indian cuisine (curry) and white mustard (yellow) is used as a condiment in the US.

RADISHES There are many types of radishes, varying in size, color and length of time they take to mature. They are generally pest and disease-free. They are easy to grow. Most varieties mature within a month. They grow best in cool weather (April to June and October to January). There are at least three glucosinoates in radishes.

3. Cyanogenic Glycosides

Have you ever wondered how Eskimos stay healthy? I was always under the impression that an Eskimo's diet consisted of blubber and fish. I wondered, "What is it that keeps them from getting sick?"

Then I read an article about plants containing Amygdalin. In the article, it listed plants that were very high in Anygdalin and one of them was tundra grass, which caribou feed on. It was also noted that caribou are the main staple of the Eskimos.

FYI: Eskimos also consider the caribou's stomach contents a delicacy–a salad of amygdalin-rich greens.

DID YOU KNOW?

QUESTION: If carnivores (mammals) only eat herbivores, then how do they stay healthy (alkaline pH) and keep from getting sick if their only food source is meat? The answer is: The first part of a *ruminant the carnivore instinctively eats is the rumen (the first stomach chamber) and/or the viscera (intestines), which contain "broken down" grasses rich in amygdalin.

Grizzly bears instinctively eat the intestines and stomach first from a fresh kill. Sometimes they eat only the grasses from the stomach and abandon the rest of the carcass. They never eat the colon.

*Ruminants are cud-chewing herbivores--cattle, deer, goats, camels, llamas, sheep, etc. who have a four-chambered stomach. Their hooves are "cloved." (Horses are not ruminants.) Ruminants swallow grasses whole, to be regurgitated later. Using the enzymes in their saliva to break down the grasses, they chew it and chew it and chew it, then re-swallow the grasses for digestion.

Sources of Cyanogenic Glycosides

Plant sources listed from the highest to the lowest. For example, apricots have the highest concentration of amygdalin and pear kernels have the lowest concentration in parts per million (ppm):

Amygdalin ($C_{20}H_{27}NO_{11}$)

Apricot (kernel), peach (leaf and kernel), plum (kernel), apple (kernel), bitter almonds, butter beans, lima beans, and pear (kernel)

Dhurrin ($C_{14}H_{17}NO_7$)

Wheat (Sprout and seedling)

Linamarin ($C_{10}H_{17}NO_6$)

Flaxseed

Linustatin ($C_{16}H_{27}NO_{11}$)

Flaxseed

Lotaustralin ($C_{11}H_{19}NO_6$)

Flaxseed

Neolinustatin ($C_{17}H_{29}NO_{11}$)

Flaxseed

Prunasin ($C_{14}H_{17}NO_6$)

Sour cherry (kernel), dandelion root, bitter almond, and peach (kernel)

Sambunigrin ($C_{14}H_{17}NO_6$)

European elderberry (leaf)

Taxiphylin ($C_{14}H_{17}NO_7$)

Common yew (leaf)

Amygdalin

Certain grasses and certain fruit kernels (peach, apricot, apple, and plum) contain anygdalin (a cyanogenic glycoside), especially the grassland grasses, which wild herbivores eat.

Several years ago, the FDA banned Laetrile, because they claimed the cyanide in Laetrile is deadly. They were right.

Laetrile ($C_{14}H_{15}NO_7$)

Laetrile is a manmade <u>manufactured</u> and <u>modified</u> form of Amygdalin, usually referred to as vitamin B17.

DID YOU KNOW?

Laetrile is <u>not</u> a vitamin. Laetrile ($C_{14}H_{15}NO_7$) and the chemical compound Amygdalin ($C_{20}H_{27}NO_{11}$) <u>do</u> <u>not</u> have the same formula. Please note the difference in their formulas.

Since Laetrile is not a "natural" cyanogenic glycoside, the cyanide molecule in Laetrile is deadly. Therefore, taking manmade Laetrile to treat cancer will cause death by cyanide.

In this chapter, I am only interested in Amygdalin, which is a cyanogenic glycoside (nitrogen-based chemical compound).

The following is WHY Amygdalin is so effective against killing cancer cells:

Amygdalin ($C_{20}H_{27}NO_{11}$)

For Anygdalin (which contains the molecules to form cyanide) to be broken down in the body, it needs the enzyme beta-glucosidase. (Remember that each enzyme is a specific key to unlock a specific door.)

FACT: The human body <u>does</u> <u>not</u> manufacture beta-glucosidase.

When the chemical compound Amygdalin is in the presence of beta-glucosidase, a chemical reaction occurs. Amygdalin is broken down into two molecules of glucose, one molecule of benzaldehyde and one molecule of hydrogen cyanide (HCN).

This is deadly for the recipient of the hydrogen cyanide, but there is a catch. Only one type of cell contains the enzyme beta-glucosidase and that is the CANCER CELL.

When the cancer cell uptakes Amygdalin, the beta-glucosidase enzyme in the cancer cell goes to work, forming the hydrogen cyanide, which KILLS the cancer cell.

Although Amygdalin does have the potential to form cyanide (CN), only the enzyme beta-glucosidase can break down Amygdalin to form the deadly hydrogen cyanide (HCN).

Since humans and other mammals <u>do</u> <u>not</u> make the enzyme beta-glucosidase and if there are no cancer cells present, cyanide is <u>never</u> released from Amygdalin and is harmlessly excreted from the body intact.

AUTHOR'S COMMENTS

If scientists emphatically state the human body's exocrine system <u>does not</u> manufacture beta-glucosidase. Then what is inside the cancer cell that is producing beta-glucosidase?

ANSWER: It could only have come from an outside source. The "what" inside the cancer cell is, of course, a pathogen—a cancer-causing microorganism that manufactures (synthesizes) beta-glucosidase.

DID YOU KNOW?

According to Wikipedia:

> "In 1977, the FDA prohibited the interstate shipment of amygdalin and laetrile. Thereafter, 27 US states legalized the use of amygdalin within those states.

Flaxseed

Flaxseeds contain four cyanogenic glycosides:

Linamarin ($C_{10}H_{17}NO_6$)

According to a reliable US government database and one other source, this alkaloid is present in the seed. However, according to Wikipedia, this cyanogenic glycoside is only in the roots and leaves of the plant.

Flaxseeds contain high levels of lignan, which are estrogen-like chemicals and act as anti-oxidants. Scientists believe lignans bind to estrogen receptors and interfere with the cancer-producing effects of estrogen on breast tissue.

Studies have shown lignans reduce the risk of breast cancer, prostate cancer and cardiovascular disease.

AUTHOR'S COMMENTS

Ground flaxseed is an excellent preventative. It can be added to food or to raw honey. The next page is a protocol that is beneficial for the eyes.

Flaxseed Protocol

You will need:

    One clean eyedropper

    Pure organic flaxseed oil (lignan-free)

Dosage:

    Two drops in each eye three times a day

Directions:

    After putting two drops in each eye, lie down and keep eyes closed for ten minutes. Dab closed eyes with clean cloth.

Author's Comments

People have reported that scar tissue has disappeared and that they did not have to wear glasses anymore after doing this protocol for several weeks.

Flaxseed Oil and Oil of Oregano Protocol

I have spent 20+ hours searching for the "missing link" in Oregano that makes it a pathogen killer. As of the publication of this book, I have not found the "missing link." However, a telltale giveaway that alkaloids are present in oil of oregano is its "bitter" taste. (Alkaloids are bitter.)

The following is an effective protocol using flaxseed and oil of oregano:

One tablespoon of organic flaxseed oil

4-6 drops oil of oregano.

Recommended dosage: Four timex a day or as needed.

AUTHOR'S COMMENTS

Not all products are created equal. Reliable sources recommend "Spectrum" organic flaxseed oil and "Soloray" or "Solgar" oil of oregano. They are available from Vitacost. (800-381-0759)

4. Sulfur

I have added sulfur as #4 on the list. Sulfur plays just as important a role as nitrogen does in a plant's defense against bacteria.

Even with all the new drugs on the market, sulfur, which has been around for a long time, is still being used to fight infections, especially urinary track infections. The following, onions, garlic and asparagus are all an excellent source of sulfur.

Onions

Onions are loaded with glucosinolates (at least 13) and other sulfur compounds (no nitrogen element attached). Onions and garlic are in the Allium family of vegetables.

Alliin ($C_6H_{11}NO_3S$)

Even though this is not a true glucosinolate, it has both nitrogen and sulfur present.

When crushing onions, the enzyme alliinase converts Alliin into Allicin. Allicin is famous for being in garlic, but it is also present in onions. Allicin is what gives garlic its potent aroma. Alliin affects immune responses in the blood.

Allicin ($C_6H_{10}OS_2$)

This is one of the plant's major defenses against attack and is derived from Alliin. It is also classified as a thiosulfinate.

DID YOU KNOW?

Some sulfur compounds give off what Wikipedia describes as a "foul" odor. These sulfur compounds are present in garlic, onions, broccoli, cabbage, and Limburger cheese (from bacterial decomposition).

These chemicals' aromas (rotting flesh and feces) are also the major attractant for blowflies and are used in baits to attract and kill disease-spreading flies.

Garlic

Garlic is a member of the Allium Family and is one of the most anti-microbial foods a person can eat. It is loaded with both sulfur and nitrogen (22 sulfur/nitrogen compounds).

Records dating back 7,000 years reveal that garlic was used as a medicinal. Even ancient Egyptians, during the building of the great pyramids, used garlic. Hippocrates and many other ancient healers mentioned garlic. The following are a few sulfur (and nitrogen) chemical compounds:

Ajoene ($C_9H_{14}OS_3$)

This sulfur-containing compound acts as an anti-oxidant Ajoene also prevents platelets in the blood from clotting, thus reducing the risk of stroke or heart disease. Studies have shown it has anti-fungal, anti-microbial and causes apoptosis.

Allicin ($C_6H_{10}OS_2$)

This gives garlic its "hot" taste. Cooking garlic diminishes allicin's potency. When garlic is chewed, damaged, or crushed, the enzyme allinase is released and converts Alliin into Allicin.

Biotin ($C_{10}H_{16}N_2O_3S$)

According to Wikipedia, diabetics may benefit from biotin. Biotin helps improve blood sugar control.

Glutathione ($C_{10}H_{17}N_3O_6S$)

This compound is a major anti-oxidant and neutralizes free radicals. Every system in the body (immune system, central nervous system, gastrointestinal system and the lungs) uses this compound. It is used in DNA synthesis and repair, amino acid transport, and enzyme activation.

The shear numbers of sulfur and nitrogen-based compounds in garlic speak for themselves. Garlic is definitely just as and more potent than onions. Some facts about garlic:

- Garlic has a reputation of making one "stinky." This is because sulfur compounds cannot be digested and are passed into the bloodstream. The compounds are then carried to the lungs and the skin, where they are excreted. Therefore, the effect of eating garlic may be present for a long time.

- Garlic helps support the "good" flora in the stomach, while killing the "bad" bacteria.
- Garlic is famous for lowering blood pressure and cholesterol levels.
- To offset garlic's odor, eat fresh parsley, which is only a short-time fix.

DID YOU KNOW?

Garlic is toxic to dogs.

Garlic and skunks have something in common. Garlic's chemical compounds and skunk spray chemicals are similar. Their sulfur compounds are "thiols."

A skunk has two glands--one on each side of its anus. These glands produce a mixture of sulfur compounds, reeking of rotten eggs, burned rubber and sulfur. A skunk can spray its enemy as far away as ten feet, but its supply of chemicals is not endless. A skunk only has enough chemicals to spray up to five or six times (does not mean in its lifetime).

Because of this defense, a skunk does not have to worry too much about land predators; BUT, because the skunk is a nocturnal critter, its only enemy is the Great Horned Owl, which hunts at night.

What amazing little stinkers garlic and skunks are -- Comrades in arms!

Asparagus

Asparagus is a cousin of onions and garlic and has many anti-cancer properties. It, too, has thiol (sulfur) compounds. Wikipedia defines thiols as "the sulfur analogues of alcohol, where sulfur takes the place of oxygen."

Methanethiol (CH_4S)

This thiol is the sulfur compound, which gives urine a strong smell 15-30 minutes after eating asparagus.

Dimethyl Disulfide ($C_2H_6S_2$)

This thiol (DMS) gives off a cabbage smell when cooked. Beets, cabbage and corn also contain DMS.

Dimethyl Sulfoxide (C_2H_6OS)

Better known as DMSO, this compound tastes like garlic. DMSO is used as a topical analgesic, because it can penetrate the skin and other membranes without damaging them, thus increasing the effectiveness of other chemical compounds (medicines). Normally used with anti-fungal medications, veterinarians use DMSO in the treatment of horses.

NOTE: The FDA has not approved DMSO for people, except for the treatment of interstitial cystitis. Surprisingly, DMSO is available over the counter.

Dimethyl Sulfone ($C_2H_6O_2S$)

This sulfur chemical compound (MSM) a/k/a $DMSO_2$ has controversy built around it.

Many health benefits have been claimed about MSM. It is sold as a dietary supplement. Books have been written about it and glucosamine sulfane. The authors claim it supports the structure and function of joints and is marketed to osteoporosis sufferers. These two are also sold with chondroitin sulfate, which is an important component of cartilage.

DID YOU KNOW?

It is against the law in the United States to market a dietary supplement as a treatment for a disease or condition.

Glutathione ($C_{10}H_{17}N_3O_6S$)

Of all the sulfur chemical compounds in asparagus, this might be the most important.

There have been many studies on this chemical compound and its anti-oxidant and anti-cancer properties. It detoxifies the cell by binding to heavy metals, solvents and pesticides.

According to the National Cancer Institute, asparagus contains more glutathione than any other food source.

Glutathione, itself, is not essential, because it consists of three amino acids: cystine, glutamic acid, and glycine. Fortunately, the body is able to manufacture (synthesize) glutathione.

Glutathione is vital for iron metabolism.

Studies have shown that there are glutathione deficiencies in people who have HIV, Alzheimer's, Parkinson's, prostate and other cancers, chronic fatigue, asthma, and physical stress. According to Wikipedia, people suffering from schizophrenia and bi-polar depression have glutathione deficiencies. Wikipedia states:

> "Glutathione helps prevent damage to cells by neutralizing harmful molecules.......also plays a role in processing medications and cancer-causing carcinogens and building DNA proteins and other important cellular components."

Glutathione is the major free radical scavenger in the brain. (This could explain why Alzheimer's victims' brains are depleted of glutathione, because the brain is under mycoplasma attack.)

Asparagus Protocol

STEP 1

Cook the asparagus

STEP 2

Puree the asparagus

STEP 3

Consume eight tablespoons twice a day (16 tablespoons = one cup)

AUTHOR'S COMMENTS

This is an excellent protocol for cancer/disease prevention. NOTE: This protocol might not be strong enough to use by itself.

This protocol can be used with an alkalizing protocol.

If you are on blood thinners, this protocol is not for you.

4. Medium-Chain Fatty Acids

Even though this, too, is not on the Wikipedia list of plant-based defense phytochemicals, I consider this an important defense against mycoplasma.

If not for people like Dr. Bruce Fife who has written many books and articles on the amazing coconut, Americans would never have learned about the coconut's super anti-microbial effect on pathogens.

FIRST, A LITTLE HISTORY

In the 1980s, a media campaign against saturated fat (coconut and palm oil) started, condemning it, saying it was bad for us. Instead, unsaturated fats, especially soybean and canola, were "pushed" on the American people, when in reality research proved these "sticky" oils are indirectly and directly related to the following:

1. Plaque buildup in the blood vessels

2. Cancer and disease

3. Damage to cells through peroxidation (more about this later)

Coconut oil is one of the most potent pathogen killers in the plant world and does not contain nitrogen! It does, however, contain some sulfur; but sulfur is not what makes it so potent. It's the medium chain fatty acids (MCFA's) found only in coconut and palm oil. The oil in coconuts is 92 percent medium chain fatty acids.

Medium chain fatty acids are also in mother's milk for a reason. The medium chain fatty acids protect the newborn from disease until the baby can build up his or her own immune system. Here's how medium chain fatty acids kill mycoplasma:

Coconut oil is not anti-microbial until the body breaks it down into monoglycerides and free fatty acids in the digestive tract. The following is from Dr. Fife's book, *Coconut Cures*:

> "Medium chain fatty acids and monoglycerides are absorbed into the organism's outer membrane. These fats have a destabilizing effect, which weakens the membrane to the point that it dissolves and falls apart, killing the organism. Bacteria cannot develop resistance to this type of action."

Studies have verified what Dr. Fife claims. Scientists have actually witnessed medium chain fatty acids dissolving mycoplasma membrane!

Dr. Fife suggests women who are nursing or who are pregnant to eat coconut oil, because coconut oil helps develop the baby's brain. He states in his book that nursing mothers who do not eat coconut oil will only provide around four percent medium chain fatty acids. But if they ingest coconut oil, medium chain fatty acids will jump to a whopping 18 percent in their milk.

There are three types of medium chain fatty acids found in coconut oil:

Lauric Acid ($C_{12}H_{24}O_2$)

According to studies, this MCFA is the most powerful of the three against mycoplasma.

Capric Acid ($C_{10}H_{20}O_2$)

This fatty acid makes up about ten percent of the medium chain fatty acids in coconut oil.

Caprylic Acid ($C_8H_{16}O_2$)

According to Wikipedia:

> "This fatty acid is used in the treatment of some bacterial infections. Due to its relatively short chain length, it has no difficulty in penetrating fatty cell wall membrane, hence its effectiveness in combating certain lipid-coated bacteria, such as Staphylococcus aureus and Streptococcus."

According to Wikipedia, this fatty acid is an anti-microbial pesticide used as a food contact surface sanitizer in commercial food handling establishments. It is used as a disinfectant in hospitals.

PEROXIDATION

Polyunsaturated (PUFA) and monounsaturated (MUFA) fatty acids require processing by pancreatic enzymes and liver bile to break them down into usable molecules.

After leaving the stomach and entering the intestinal tract, long chain fatty acids are broken down into lipoproteins. After processing, the lipoproteins are absorbed through the intestinal walls into the bloodstream and begin circulating. As the lipoproteins circulate, fat is released. There has been much research about unsaturated fat and peroxidation. The following is Wikipedia's definition of lipid peroxidation:

> "Lipid peroxidation refers to the oxidative degradation of lipids. It is the process in which free radicals steal elements

from the lipids in cell membranes resulting in cell damage. This process proceeds by a free radical chain reaction mechanism. It most often affects polyunsaturated fatty acids. If not terminated fast enough, there will be damage to the cell membrane, which consists mainly of lipids. In addition, end-products of lipid peroxidation may be mutagenic and carcinogenic."

Did you notice the word polyunsaturated? Both Dr. Bruce Fife and Dr. Raymond Peat (another coconut advocate) state polyunsaturated fats are unhealthy and damage cell walls.

We have been fed "big fat lies" for years. It should be simple to connect the dots, as to why mycoplasma can easily penetrate "damaged" cell walls (made of processed polyunsaturated fats).

According to Wikipedia:

"Polyunsaturated fat can be found mostly in nuts, seeds, fish, algae, leafy greens and krill. Whole food sources are best. Processing and heating may damage polyunsaturated fats."

The following is a list of polyunsaturated fat (oil) that will boggle your mind: Walnut Oil; Sunflower Oil; Sesame Seed Oil; Corn Oil; Flaxseed Oil; Safflower Oil; Canola (Rapeseed) Oil; Cottonseed Oil; Peanut Oil; Olive Oil (25% polyunsaturated); and Soybean Oil.

Based on Wikipedia's excerpt, the more processed the seed, the more it can turn rancid (peroxidation).

Monounsaturated fats have less chance of turning rancid because they have one double bond in their fatty chain, whereas polyunsaturated fats have more than one double bond in their fatty acid chain.

According to Wikipedia, "Monounsaturated fat is found in red meat, whole milk, nuts, olives, avocados, peanuts, macadamia nuts, almonds, sunflowers, sesame seeds, whole grain wheat, and oatmeal.

Many of the above oils have a combination of both polyunsaturated and monounsaturated. For example, olive oil is 75% monounsaturated fat, and cashews are 58% monounsaturated fat.

According to *Coconut Oil-Arthritis*, an article written by Dr. Raymond Peat, general aging and especially aging of the brain are associated with lipid peroxidation.

Polyunsaturated fats are used as paint-stock oils because they are "sticky." These include safflower, corn, soy and linseed (flaxseed). "Sticky" polyunsaturated fat helps paint adhere to the surface.

Dr. Peat makes an interesting point in his article entitled *Coconut Oil-Arthritis*. "Lesions in blood vessels are caused by lipid peroxidation of unsaturated oils and relate to <u>stress</u> because <u>adrenaline</u> liberates fat from storage."

THE THYROID GLAND

There are even more benefits from eating coconut oil. Did you know (according to Dr. Raymond Peat) that unsaturated fat <u>suppresses</u> the metabolic rate? Dr. Peat states unsaturated oil specifically suppresses tissue response to thyroid hormone and the transport of hormones.

Dr. Peat makes a very intelligent point that seeds have built-in chemical defenses that can block digestive enzymes in the stomach. He also states that the thyroid gland uses an enzyme to make hormones and that <u>unsaturated fat inhibits</u> the thyroid enzyme. He further states coconut oil supports thyroid function and <u>the thyroid determines brain development</u>.

Dr. Peat stated the suppression of the thyroid gland raises serum cholesterol. He explains that a 1930s study revealed when the thyroid gland is functioning properly and producing hormones, there will be no excess cholesterol in the blood. (FYI: Cholesterol is the main component of hormones.) Low thyroid function causes:

    1. Digestion to slow down

    2. Healing to slow down

    3. Immune response to slow down

    4. Hormone and enzyme production to slow down

    5. Body temperature to drop

Some symptoms of low thyroid are:

    A. Overweight (hypothyroid)

    B. Cold hands and feet

    C. Fatigue

    D. Swelling

    E. Low libido

    F. Irregular menstrual periods (women)

It is interesting to point out that the above symptoms can also be associated with a mycoplasma infection.

Mycoplasma can wreak havoc on the endocrine system, and the thyroid gland is part of the endocrine system. Wikipedia's definition of the endocrine system is:

> "The endocrine system is made up of a series of glands that produce chemicals called hormones."

The main ingredient of a hormone is fat. Hormones regulate everything--sleep (melatonin), mood (dopamine), intake of glucose and lipids (insulin), and cognition (dopamine), just to name a few.

Other endocrine system organs and their glands, which produce hormones are: Head/Brain/Neck (hypothalamus, pineal gland, pituitary gland thyroid gland); Liver; Kidney; Duodenum; Pancreas; Stomach; Adrenal Gland; Ovaries; Testes (male); Placenta and Uterus (when a woman is pregnant); Skin; Parathyroid; Heart; Bone Marrow; and Adipose Tissue

Wikipedia states the hypothalamus controls body temperature, hunger, thirst, fatigue, motor control, mood (depression), and sleep.

WEIGHT LOSS AND COCONUT OIL

In Dr. Fife's book, he states that coconut oil raises the metabolic rate (burn more calories) because coconut oil is immediately used for fuel. Coconut oil makes a person feel "full," which lasts for several hours. Studies have shown people eat less when supplementing their diet with coconut oil.

SKIN CARE AND COCONUT OIL

Coconut oil, when both applied topically and ingested, rejuvenates the skin.

COCONUT OIL NUTRITION

Studies have shown that coconut oil improves vitamin and mineral absorption. Not only does it enhance the B vitamins but also D, E and K, as well as beta-carotene (A). It also helps maximize mineral absorption (magnesium and calcium). Coconut oil contains iron, sodium, and zinc.

COCONUT WATER

In Hawaii, the natives call coconut water Noelani, which translates to "dew from the heavens."

Coconut water is obtained from green coconuts. Green coconuts are not ripe. (If you would drink the water from a ripe coconut it would taste sour.)

Since coconut tree roots derive their water source from the ocean, coconut water is rich with oceanic minerals, such as potassium, magnesium and calcium. Dr. Fife states that an eight-ounce glass of coconut water has more potassium in it than a banana.

Although coconut meat is rich in saturated oils, coconut water's fat content is very low. Its sugar content is low, too.

According to Dr. Fife, coconut water contains more essential electrolytes than over-the-counter sports drink. Wikipedia's description of electrolytes is as follows:

> "....the primary ions of electrolytes are sodium (Na^+), potassium (K^+), magnesium (Mg^{2+}), chloride (Cl^-), hydrogen carbonate (HCO_3^-) and hydrogen phosphate (HPO_4^{2-}), Without sufficient levels of these key electrolytes, muscle weakness or severe muscle contractions may occur."

According to an article written by Dr. Bruce Fife entitled *Coconut Water: Dew from the Heavens*, coconut water helps dilate blood vessels, improves blood flow, and reduces plaque formation.

Cytokinins

Coconut water contains a plant growth hormone called cytokinin. This hormone is said to be anti-aging. According to Wikipedia, Folkee Skoog discovered the effects of cytokinins in coconut water in the 1940s.

In plants, cytokinins are involved in cell division and growth and influence the rate at which plants age. Cytokinins in plants are similar to human growth hormones called cytokines. According to Dr. Fife, the amount of cytokinins present can determine the aging of the plant to accelerate or slow down. He states plants deprived of cytokinins age faster than normal. He also states that cytokinins have an anti-aging effect on human cells!

The following is a quote borrowed from Dr. Fife's article on the benefits of drinking coconut water:

> "Treated cells never undergo the severe degenerative changes experienced by untreated cells........reducing risk of developing degenerative and age-related diseases."

AUTHOR'S COMMENTS

Could ingesting coconut oil and drinking coconut water reduce the risk of age-related macular degeneration? FACT: In 2014 there were eight million people in the US diagnosed with age-related macular degeneration. Today, 2016, there are over eleven million diagnosed cases of age-related macular degeneration. I believe macular diseases are caused by "degenerative" maculas which are vulnerable to bacterial attack. (The macula consists of fat and mycoplasma needs fat!) What do you think?

Coconut water should not be confused with coconut milk. They are entirely different. Coconut water is only found in "green" coconuts, whereas coconut milk is made from the grated meat of the coconut.

Coconut oil is effective against the following bacteria:

<u>Streptococcus</u> Some of these bacteria are pathogenic and some are nonpathogenic. One member of Streptococci is a necessary component in the production of Swiss cheese.

<u>E-coli</u> Escherichia coli are a rod-shaped bacteria group found in the lower intestines of warm-blooded animals. Most e-coli are harmless but some can cause serious food poisoning.

<u>Chlamydia</u> There are three bacteria classified as Chlamydia. (See The Truth about Heart Disease chapter, page 47.)

<u>Staphylococcus</u> (Staph) colonizes the skin and upper respiratory tract of mammals and birds.

<u>Methicillin-resistant Staphylococcus aureus</u> (MRSA) is responsible for serious difficult-to-treat infections in humans and has developed a resistance to antibiotics. Hospitals fear this pathogen, which colonizes in the host's nostrils

According to *Coconut Cures*, coconut oil (MCFA) also kills viruses:

<u>Measles</u> Measles is an infection of the respiratory tract that is caused by the paramyxovirus. It is spread by an infected person's coughing and sneezing (aerosol) and is very contagious.

<u>Herpes Simplex</u> Oral herpes referred to as a cold sore or fever blister. Genital herpes is the second most common form of herpes.

Section 6

"Killing" Pathogens

Tobacco

The tobacco (Nicotiana) plant is in the family of Nightshade. Of all the Nightshade plants available medicinally, tobacco is in the top ten plant list with the highest concentration of alkaloids. The tobacco plant is very toxic and deadly if ingested.

FYI: The plant itself has +60 alkaloids. Five percent of the leaf consists of alkaloids plus many other nitrogen-based chemical compounds, which are not classified as alkaloids.

NICOTINE ($C_{10}H_{14}N_2$)

Nicotine is the alkaloid people associate with the word tobacco. Used as a pesticide, it acts as a neurotoxin to insects. Nicotine paralyzes and kills insects by interfering with the transmitter substance between nerves and muscles.

AMMONIA (NH_3)

Ammonia is present naturally in the tobacco plant. Ammonia is a natural antiseptic (anti-microbial) compound. In the movie *Food, Inc.* the fast food beef processing industry disinfects hamburger with ammonia. They claim disinfecting (washing) hamburger in ammonia reduces the e-Coli bacteria to undetectable levels.

There have been many studies done using the nicotine patch--Parkinson's, ADD/HD, schizophrenia, Irritable Bowel Syndrome, and depression; and they all have shown benefits from the nicotine patch.

There was an interesting study published in *Neurology* in 2011. The study involved Alzheimer's patients (mild cognitive impairment). Half the participants wore a 15-mg nicotine patch, and the other half wore a placebo. At the end of the six-month study, the patients who wore a nicotine patch--their health improved and their memory improved. The ones who wore the placebo--their health worsened.

Nicotine in the patch *is* not acting alone in killing microorganisms, because there are over 60 other nitrogen-based phytochemicals in tobacco.

The tobacco plant depletes the soil of minerals and nutrients.

Wearing multiple patches (totaling over 30 mg) can be lethal. Signs of poisoning are dizziness and vomiting.

DANGER: Keep nicotine patches away from pregnant women, children and pets.

Marijuana (Hemp)

Much controversy over using the marijuana plant for medicinal purposes has occurred in the last 60+ years. The main controversy has been over a chemical compound found in the buds of the marijuana (hemp) plant–THC.

THC ($C_{21}H_{30}O_2$)

Tetrahydrocannabinol (a cannabinoid), also known as delta-9-tetrahydrocannabinol, is present on the flowers and buds of the cannabis (marijuana) plant.

Researchers claim THC is one of the most powerful and effective treatments for disease and cancer ever discovered by man.

THC is actually a phenol. Phenols are another type of chemical defense a plant uses to defend itself from insects and herbivores. Phenols are the source for the plant's flavor and/or aroma.

Even 5,000 years ago, there is evidence that the ancient Chinese used cannabis as a medicinal. Up until the early 1900s, holistic doctors were prescribing and using cannabis to treat disease. This was standard practice until allopathic medicine took control of the medical industry.

In 1942, cannabis was removed from the Pharmacopoeia, which is a reference for pharmaceutical drug preparation.

Then in 1970, the government (under the Controlled Substance Act) placed cannabis into the Schedule 1 category. (Schedule 1 is the only category of controlled substances that absolutely <u>may not</u> be prescribed by a physician.)

A drug must meet <u>all three</u> of the following criteria to be placed in the Schedule 1 category:

1. The drug or other substance has a high potential for abuse.

2. The drug or other substance has no currently accepted medical use in treatment in the US.

3. There is a lack of accepted safety for use of the drug or other substance under medical supervision.

AUTHOR'S COMMENT

FYI: The FDA and the DEA are the only Federal agencies that can add or remove a substance from the schedules (Schedule 1-5).

If our government classified cannabis as a Schedule 1 drug and banned it, why is the Health and Human Services Division of the Federal government the holder of US patent #6,630,507 for medical cannabis?

This patent is entitled "Cannabinoids as Anti-oxidants and Neuroprotectorants," and is dated October 7, 2003. It reads in part:

> "Cannabinoids have been found to have antioxidant properties, unrelated to NMDA receptor antagonism. This new found property makes cannabinoids useful in the treatment and prophylaxis of wide variety of oxidation associated diseases such as ischemic, age-related, inflammatory, and autoimmune diseases. The cannabinoids are found to have particular application as neuro-protectorants, for example in limiting neurological damage, following ischemic insults such as stroke and trauma, or in the treatment of neurodegenerative diseases, such as Alzheimer's disease, Parkinson's disease and HIV dementia......"

RICK SIMPSON'S STORY

Rick Simpson of Nova Scotia, Canada, heard about the medicinal value of the cannabis Indica plant when he, himself had skin cancer. According to his testimony, after treating himself for only four days topically with the oil, his skin cancer disappeared.

He knew that the growing of cannabis in Canada was illegal but went ahead and grew it on his property for other cancer patients. He has treated over 1,000 people diagnosed with cancer (some with terminal cancer).

Unfortunately, the Canadian government stepped in and he was charged with trafficking and the possession of an illegal substance, even though he didn't charge anyone for the treatment(s).

In 2007, he stood before the Canadian Supreme court and was found guilty.

However, his legacy lives on. He is still crusading for people to have the right to receive cannabis treatments. His story/documentary *Run from the Cure* is on youTube. Visit his web site:

www.phoenixtears.ca

There are three types of cannabis (marijuana) plants:

- Sativa (Indian hemp) grows very tall and slender

- Indica is shorter than Sativa and is bushy (this is the plant Rick Simpson grew)
- Ruderalis is the shortest of the three and is slender

Scientists are still mystified as to why THC is so effective against cancer and disease. Studies have shown that THC is just that—effective against cancer and disease.

According to Rick Simpson, he extracted pure THC from the plants' buds and did not use the leaves or stalks.

He also claims the cannabis Indica plant produces the best quality and most potent THC.

The following are some findings (claims) from scientific studies on THC's effectiveness against cancer and disease:

- THC relieves inflammation and pain (including neuopathic pain).
- THC has been proven to be effective against Crohn's disease.
- THC relieves the symptoms of rheumatoid arthritis, depression, insomnia, lupus, and fibromyalgia
- THC has an anti-tumoral effect, which means it counteracts or prevents the formation of malignant tumors.
- THC is anti-mitogenic, meaning that it inhibits cancer cell division.
- THC is pro-apoptotic, meaning THC encourages the process of programmed cell death (PCD).
- THC has been shown to be very effective against lung cancer, which is normally aggressive and resistant to chemotherapy. (FYI: Cancer is the #2 leading cause of death in the USA and lung cancer claims the lives of 160,000 people a year.)
- THC inhibits metastasis. (Metastasis means that the cancer cells spread, usually through the bloodstream to another organ or location in the body.)
- THC is anti-angiogenic, which means that it interferes with the growth of new blood vessels to the cancer cells.

US Patent on THC

To read about the US patent on cannabinoids, go to Wikipedia and type into their search engine "Cannabinoid," then scroll down the page to the US Patent no. 6630507.

To view the patent, search "medical cannabis" and scroll down the page to 10.9 United States where you can view and read the entire patent.

The next chapter reveals the "real" truth about marijuana and proves that THC is a just a "smokescreen."

The Truth about Marijuana

The cannabis plant, seeds and root contain over 480 chemical compounds. These include nitrogen-based compounds, terpenes, and phenols.

THC ($C_{21}H_{30}O_2$)

Scientists and researchers claim it is THC that is the anti-cancer agent in cannabis.

FACT: Only **nitrogen-based** and **nitrogen/sulfur-based** chemical compounds have the potential to **kill** pathogens.

Notice THC's chemical formula is Cs, Hs and Os. THC is not an alkaloid and there is <u>no</u> nitrogen or sulfur present in the formula. Further, THC is a <u>phenol</u>, which is associated with "aroma" or "flavor." THC is the chemical compound in the marijuana plant that is responsible for the user's "high."

MARIJUANA ALKALOIDS

Scientific studies have documented alkaloids present in cannabis (hemp). In my search for the truth, I did find at least <u>ten</u> (along with other nitrogen-based compounds) present in either the root or the plant itself. I suspect there are many more yet to be discovered. The following are <u>documented</u> alkaloids present in cannabis:

Neurine ($C_5H_{13}NO$)

This is an interesting alkaloid. Considered poisonous, it is in egg yolk, brain bile and <u>cadavers</u>.

It is formed during the purification (breaking down of the cells) of tissues by the dehydration of choline. Neurine has a "fishy" odor.

Trigonelline ($C_7H_7NO_2$)

This alkaloid is in the seeds of cannabis. It is also found in fenugreek seed, coffee beans, garden peas, oats and potatoes. Studies have shown that trigonelline is anti-cancer (cervix and liver), anti-tumor (cervix and liver), and is a natural insecticide.

Atropine ($C_{17}H_{23}NO_3$)

This alkaloid is present in the <u>root</u> of the cannabis plant. According to Wikipedia, Atropine is used as an antidote for insecticide and nerve gas poisoning. Military troops who are under threat of chemical weapon attack carry auto injectors of atropine and obidoxine, which can quickly be injected in the thigh. (Atropine is in the auto injector because it slows down the action of the nerve gas or other poison, giving obidoxine time to work.)

Atropine is used as an antidote for a black widow spider bite and the ingestion of poison mushrooms.

Some of the side effects of atropine are: ventricular fibrillation, dizziness, blurred vision, loss of balance, dry mouth, dilated pupils, and confusion.

Hordenine ($C_{10}H_{15}NO$)

In mammals, this alkaloid works as a stimulant, meaning it increases heart rate and blood pressure and stimulates the release of norepinephrine.

Piperidine ($C_5H_{11}N$)

Classified as an amine, Piperidine is a "base" for several alkaloids, including piperine found in black pepper. It is the base for the fire ant's poison and the poisonous hemlock's alkaloid conine. This amine is the building block in the manufacturing of many pharmaceutical drugs such as PCP (angel dust).

Muscarine ($C_9H_{20}NO_2^+$)

This is a potent alkaloid. Muscarine derivatives are used in the treatment of glaucoma. According to Wikipedia, muscarine can powerfully stimulate the muscular fiber in the intestines, the secretion of the pancreas, liver, and intestinal mucous membranes.

Muscarine poisoning is usually associated with the ingesting of poison mushrooms, which contain muscarine.

Cannabinine

Discovered and named in the 1800s, this alkaloid is present in the marijuana plant.

Anhydrocannabisativine

A recent study isolated and named this alkaloid, which is in both the <u>leaves</u> and the <u>root</u> of Indian hemp (Cannabis Sativa).

Cannabisativine

Another recent study isolated this alkaloid from the root of the Indian hemp plant (Cannabis Sativa).

Isocannabisativine

This alkaloid is in the root.

CONCLUSION

It is definitely the alkaloids in cannabis and not THC that make marijuana anti-cancer and anti-disease. Until scientists and doctors "see the light," they will remain "high" on THC.

The following chapter is an amazing and uplifting story of a woman, who discovered an innovative way to use marijuana, which is benefiting people around the world. She calls her product, Hemp-EaZE™, "Healing at the Root of the Problem."

The Story of Hemp-EaZe™

Over fourteen years ago, Darcy Stoddard began a journey. It started with what she refers to as "a quick fall." This fall dislocated her ankle, shattered three inches of leg bone, shredded her tendons and severed the nerves, which required extensive surgery.

In her story, she states that a year after surgery, her ankle was still swollen and she was in constant pain. She could not walk more than five minutes and her foot was always numb.

Disheartened by her doctor's prognosis that she should get used to using a cane and take cortisone for the swelling, she lost confidence in allopathic medicine. That is when she decided to change course–she would seek and find an alternative remedy herself.

Fortunately, most of her life she had been learning what she calls the "Ancient ways" of healing herbs and the medicinal use of them. For over thirty years, she had been making salves from herbs for her family's minor aches and pains that she had grown in her own garden.

While seeking the "right" herbs for a topical cream, she had the good fortune of running into an operator/owner of a cannabis coalition, who suggested she try cannabis root. The operator said that cannabis root reduced swelling and eased pain.

Fascinated, Darcy began her research. Unfortunately, the only information she could find was a mention of an old Appalachian remedy that used hemp root for arthritis and pain.

Darcy had already chosen eight herbs to be in her cream and added the hemp root, making it a nine-herb formula. (FYI: In her story she states the eight herbs are: Comfrey, Burdock, Hyssop, Sage, Lavender, Lobelia, California Bay, and Myrrh Gum.)

When applied, the cream instantly soothed the pain. Amazingly, after only two months of applying the cream to her ankle, the swelling was completely gone and the pain was less frequent.

Then after one year of applying the cream, she regained full movement of her ankle and full feeling had come back in her leg all the way down to her toes. Lastly, the pain was gone.

Her family and friends were amazed by what she had discovered and they wanted to try it, too. Incredibly, they started getting relief from arthritis and sore muscles, and the word started spreading.

She was encouraged to market her cream, but she was hesitant—wanting to be sure it really worked. So for three years, she test marketed it (all across the country) with people suffering from arthritis, people receiving chemo, and people suffering from old and new injuries.

The results were a success. People reported that her cream relieved painful scar tissue, sprains, broken toes, psoriasis and fibromyalgia.

It was only after receiving this positive feedback that she decided to put it on the market. She called it Hemp-EaZe, which means "healing at the root of the problem."

Along the way, she learned of another important fact—the marijuana root in Hemp-EaZe contained <u>no</u> THC, which meant no "high."

More importantly, Hemp-EaZe was exempt from the Federal Substance Abuse Act, because it was suspended in oils and waxes and is not consumed (ingested).

Darcy's company uses certified organic food standard guidelines when preparing Hemp-EaZe products, meaning there are no chemicals or toxins in the formula. She states this ensures quality. To learn more about this wonderful discovery or to purchase Hemp-EaZe, visit Darcy's web site(s):

www.tierrasolfarm.com

www.hemp-eaze.com

Hemp Seeds

Commercially sold hemp seeds are from the medicinal cannabis plant Sativa, also known as Indian hemp.

This seed is incredible--I rate it one of the top super foods available to man. Hemp seeds are high in protein, containing <u>all</u> eight essential amino acids.

FYI: The human body needs 21 amino acids to function properly. The hemp seed is the only plant source, which contains the first ten amino acids necessary to stay healthy.

Edestin ($C_{32}H_{39}NO_2$)

This important amino acid is a globulin amino acid. The definition of globulin is:

> O<u>ne</u> of the <u>three</u> types of proteins (globulin, albumin and fibrinogen) found in serum, i.e., blood plasma.

The human body uses globulins as building blocks to manufacture many things, including enzymes, hemoglobin, antibodies, DNA and hormones.

The hemp seed also contains albumin protein. According to Wikipedia:

> "Albumin protein makes up 60 percent of the human blood plasma proteins."

Albumin proteins regulate blood volume and act as "taxi cabs," meaning they are carriers of molecules such as nutrients, minerals, and vitamins.

Methionine ($C_5H_{11}NO_2S$)

This essential amino acid helps protect the liver. It is also found in other seeds, such as sunflower, Brazil nuts, sesame, fenugreek, pumpkin, watermelon, soybean, poppy seed, barley, oats, and wheat.

IMPORTANCE OF ESSENTIAL FATTY ACIDS

Cell walls are 87% fat. The brain is 75% fat. Myelin sheath (fat) wraps and protects the nerve cells. Essential fatty acids (EFAs) are fats the body cannot manufacture. They must be ingested. They are omega-3 fatty acids and omega-6 fatty acids. Hemp seed is loaded with omega-3 and omega-6 fatty acids.

Ideally, for the human body to sustain proper health, both essential fatty acids should be ingested together, because the body uses them in conjunction with each other. Good news–hemp seed contains both.

Linoleic Acid ($C_{18}H_{32}O_2$)

This essential fatty acid is an omega-6 fatty acid. It is in <u>cell</u> <u>membrane</u>. A deficiency in omega-6 EFAs can result in loss of hair, poor circulation, gallbladder problems, inflammation of the prostate, slow wound healing, and growth retardation (in children).

Good sources of omega-6 EFAs: English walnuts, avocados, sunflower seeds, Brazil nuts, sesame seeds, poppy seeds, hemp seeds, pumpkin seeds, peanuts, strawberry seeds, soybeans, and chia seeds.

gamma-Linolenic Acid ($C_{18}H_{30}O_2$)

This is another omega-6 (GLA) essential fatty acid in hemp seed. The body manufactures GLA from linoleic acid.

alpha-Linolenic Acid ($C_{18}H_{30}O_2$)

This essential amino acid is an omega-3 EFA. It is also an isomer of gamma-Linolenic Acid. (An isomer has the same amount and the same elements of another molecule, except the elements are arranged differently.)

Stearidonic Acid ($C_{18}H_{28}O_2$)

This omega-3 fatty acid can be biosynthesized by the body from alpha-Linolenic acid. It naturally occurs in hemp seed. According to one source, the body converts Stearidonic Acid and gamma-Linolenic Acid into polyunsaturated (PUFA) fatty acids. PUFAs are needed by the brain to perform properly, i.e., perception, cognition, memory, vision and behavior.

Deficiencies in omega-3 EFAs can result in dry skin, high blood pressure, impaired vision, immune system dysfunction, low metabolism and poor motor coordination.

The benefits of ingesting hemp seeds are:

- Increases calcium absorption in the bones
- Reduces calcium loss from excretion
- Increases blood circulation
- Helps regulate cholesterol

- Promotes healing

The hemp plant does not accumulate toxins, as do other sources of protein (animals) that store toxic residues in their flesh. Thus, supplementing your diet with hemp seeds will reduce the risk of building up toxic chemicals in human tissues.

Trigonelline ($C_7H_7NO_2$)

This alkaloid is found in the seeds of cannabis.

Cat's Claw

Cat's Claw (Una de Gato) grows in the tropical forests of Central and South America. Used medicinally for over two thousand years, the plant gets its name from its claw-shaped thorns. The parts of this woody vine that are used medicinally are the inner bark and root.

It is used to treat intestinal ailments (Crohn's, ulcers and tumors), parasites, and colitis.

I documented eleven alkaloids.

AUTHOR'S COMMENTS

As you can see, this herbal remedy is super anti-microbial, and there is a bonus--Cat's Claw enhances the immune system.

Oleander

Referred to in the Bible as the "Desert Rose," Oleander has been used as a medicinal as far back as 3500 years ago. The leaves eaten raw are deadly, but if processed correctly as an extract, it is highly potent and kills pathogens.

Dr. H. Zima Ozel is responsible for bringing oleander to the world's attention. In 1966, he happened upon a Turkish village where he observed the inhabitants were healthy and disease-free compared to other villages. Being naturally curious, he discovered they were all taking an ancient folk remedy used for over 2,000 years.

Using the same formula, Dr. Ozel began producing his own medicinal, calling it Anvirzel®. He has been using this formula for over forty years to treat cancer and other diseases, but, unfortunately, his product is only available outside of the United States.

Dr. Ozel made a mistake. He claimed his treatment "cured" cancer, and that kept it from being FDA-approved, which would have made it available in the USA.

His product did pass FDA phase 1 trials, but because of the cost, no further attempts to get it approved for use in the USA were made.

Surprisingly, it is available in the United States under a different name and manufactured by a different company. Sold as a supplement and not as a "drug," the name of the supplement (capsules) is Utopia Natural Rose Laurel OPC Plus and is available at:

www.utopiasilver.com

For those who are interested in growing and making their own oleander extract, Tony Isaacs has written an e-book on the amazing facts and how-to's on this plant. His "oleander soup" recipe is the "real deal" and he has other cancer-fighting tips on his web site:

www.tbyil.com/anticancer.htm

WARNING: Ingesting raw oleander is deadly. If you decide to grow oleander and process it yourself, carefully follow the "oleander soup" instructions.

AUTHOR'S COMMENTS

Now, this is what I enjoy most--to uncover "the truth" as to why oleander is so effective against pathogens.

First, scientists are "stuck" on the cardiac glycoside (polysaccharides) chemical compounds in Oleander. Yes, they might have good reason–research has shown they affect the heart.

I documented nine long chain polysaccharides in Oleander: (Their formulas are all Cs, Hs and Os.) You might be wondering why I am emphasizing "long-chain polysaccharides." (Saccharide is a sugar.)

FACT: Mycoplasma builds its membrane (cell wall) out of lipids (fat) and long-chain polysaccharides.

I then searched for Oleander alkaloids and came up with only one:

Oleandomycin ($C_{35}H_{61}NO_{12}$)

This is when I asked myself, "There's got to be more. This plant is deadly. If not alkaloids, then what is in oleander that is so effective in killing mycoplasma?" HINT: it is not the long-chain polysaccharides.

Not giving up, I researched Oleander's family, because, again, family members share alkaloids.

During my search for the missing link, I had another OMG moment– Oleander and Vinca Minor (myrtle) are in the same family (Apocynaceae), and Myrtle alone has over 50 documented alkaloids!

CONCLUSION

The Biblical "Desert Rose" extract is potent against cancer and disease-causing pathogens, especially mycoplasma.

FACT: Scientists have yet to discover ALL the alkaloids in plants such as marijuana, cinnamon, turmeric, ginger and oleander.

THEORY: When mycoplasma uptakes oleander's long-chain polysaccharides to use for replication, it gets a big dose of Oleander's deadly alkaloids, resulting in the death of the mycoplasna.

Wasn't Mother Nature clever when she put long-chain polysaccharides (and alkaloids) in a plant--just for a mycoplasma's benefit?

Vinca Minor

If someday we lose our "medical freedom," this is an excellent "home remedy" if other protocols are unavailable or outlawed.

Vinca minor is also known as periwinkle or myrtle. It is in the same family with oleander.

Vinca minor contains at least 50 alkaloids in the leaves, stems and root. It is one of the top five plants with the highest concentrations of alkaloids

In all probability, like oleander, the vinca minor plant is poisonous if ingested; but alkaloids can be extracted from vinca minor's stems and leaves.

If you have a house with a yard, grow vinca minor. It is a very pretty ground cover. It might take a couple of years to establish, but it will be worth it. You will have your own medicine growing right in your own yard.

On the next page is the protocol, which I have put together and used myself. It works but takes several weeks to see results.)

Vinca Minor Protocol

You will need:

- Stainless steel cooking pot with lid (holds around a gallon of water)
- An empty clean one-gallon jug (if plastic, no BPA)
- Colander
- Paper towels
- Funnel
- A large mixing bowl
- Scissors

Materials:

- One gallon distilled or purified water
- Vinca minor stems and leaves (enough to fill cooking pot)

DIRECTIONS:

Cut vinca minor vines from plant. Do not cut (scalp) plant to the ground. Leave enough so that it will grow back. Cut enough to fill cooking pot.

Rinse leaves and stems. Put stems and leaves in pot. With scissors, cut up leaves and stems so inside the leaves/stems are exposed. (Do not use a juicer—this would be disastrous.) Cutting the stems and leaves allows the alkaloids to escape easier.

Pour distilled water into pot and bring to a boil. Boil for approximately ten minutes. Turn burner down to where water is just below the boiling stage (steeping). Put lid on pot and let steep for several hours. Occasionally stir. NOTE: The water will turn a brownish color and the leaves will darken.

When done, let stand another hour to cool.

Pour liquid (with stems and leaves) through colander into large bowl. Press leaves and stems (in the colander) to squeeze out liquid. Discard leaves and stems.

Put paper towels in colander. Using colander with paper towels (as a filter), pour liquid through the colander back into the cooking pot. (The paper towels trap debris that the colander allowed to pass through.)

NOTE: You might have to replace paper towels during this step, as debris will clog up the paper towels, not allowing liquid to pass through.

When satisfied that debris is removed, use funnel to pour liquid into gallon jug. Let cool before refrigerating.

AUTHOR'S COMMENTS

I did not get this protocol out of a book or on the web. I created the formula and experimented on myself. I started off with a teaspoon. Then, I gradually upped the dosage. Finally I was up to six shots three times a day.

Once I got used to the taste, I drank it straight–not mixing anything with it. The decoction (see Essiac tea for explanation of decoction) tasted "bitter" but this is what alkaloids taste like–bitter. My slogan is, "The more bitter, the better."

WARNING: This protocol has not been tested on children, pregnant women or pets.

AUTHOR'S COMMENTS

We are steadily losing our medical freedom and may have no other choice but to use remedies that we have grown ourselves.

This protocol might take at least one month to show results, unlike a mild silver protein IV, which "knocks out" fungus, mycoplasma, Lyme and other pathogenic microorganisms quickly and effectively.

The plant in the next chapter is considered the "king of all herbs," which can kill viruses.

Goldenseal

Goldenseal is also known as orangeroot or yellow puccoon. It is in the buttercup family Goldenseal is native to southeastern Canada and the eastern United States. As in many other medicinal plants such as bloodroot, the potent alkaloids are located in the rhizome and the roots.

Goldenseal was very popular in the mid 1800s. Native American Indians used Goldenseal as a cancer treatment.

Goldenseal is in the top five plants with the highest concentration of alkaloids. One of the potent alkaloids in Goldenseal is berberine.

AUTHOR'S COMMENTS

Based on my own experience, Goldenseal kills viruses. I have had Human Parvo B19 five times (I am in that 20% group that keeps getting it back). The last time I had a flare up, I used Goldenseal and within a month the Human Parvo virus had either died or gone back into remission. The following is a description of what an alkaloid can do:

> Alkaloids can affect cell membrane and cytoskeletal (the cell's "skeleton," which is located inside the cell and is made of protein) structure causing the cells to weaken, collapse, and affect nerve transmission.

The phrase "made of protein" is a clue as to why alkaloids can be effective against a virus. (Viruses are encased in protein.)

Walmart has its own brand of herbals under the name Spring Valley. Goldenseal is available at Walmart under that brand. Unfortunately, not all Walmarts carry Goldenseal. Check with the pharmacy and they can order it. As of November 2016, one bottle cost $5.99 for 40 capsules. (This is very reasonable.)

Goldenseal comes in extract, tincture and capsules. I prefer the non-alcohol extract and the capsules, depending on circumstances.

WARNING: Pregnant women and children should not take Goldenseal.

Marigold

Have you ever wondered why rabbits will not cross a perimeter of marigolds around your garden? The rabbits sense something our ancestors knew, that marigolds are a natural barrier--a pesticide and a natural remedy against disease and cancer.

The marigold plant contains nitrogen-based phytochemicals and is the second highest documented alkaloid-rich plant, right after the #1 poppy (opium). Twenty percent of the parts per million in this plant are alkaloids (190,000 ppm).

According to Wikipedia, the flowers were used by ancient Greek, Roman, Middle Eastern and Indian cultures as a medicinal herb, as well as a dye for fabric and cosmetics. Flowers also contain leutin, and lycopene.

This is an important garden plant that pharmacological studies show to be anti-viral. Unlike oleander or vinca minor the plant is edible.

This is another plant you can grow easily yourself for medicinal purposes.

To make the marigold protocol, use the vinca minor protocol on page 145.

Essiac Tea

René Caisse was the third daughter in a family of eleven children and was born on August 11, 1888, in Bracebridge, Canada.

She pursued a career in nursing and in 1922, while working as a head nurse in a hospital, she observed an elderly woman with a mass of breast scar tissue being bathed. The woman told her of being cured of breast cancer 50 years previously by an herbal remedy used by the native Indian people of northern Ontario.

Convinced that the medicinal remedy had value, for two years she experimented, tested and refined the mixture of burdock root, sheep sorrel, slippery elm bark and Turkish rhubarb root. She used her mother's basement as her laboratory and experimented on mice.

She named the brew Essiac, which was her family name spelled backwards. At that time, she felt confident enough to try it out on her first patient. Her first patient was her aunt who had been given only six months to live. Because of the law, she had to get her aunt's doctor's permission to administer it under his supervision. Her aunt recovered and lived another 25 years.

Other cases, which had failed to respond to other medical treatments were referred to her by the same doctor. Word of mouth spread of the miraculous recoveries due to Essiac and more doctors referred cancer patients to her. After working all day at the hospital, René treated up to thirty patients every evening after work.

It was at that time that she decided to give up her nursing career and pursue giving the treatment full-time. Since this wasn't officially proved a treatment by the medical establishment, she did not charge her patients for treatments.

Without an income, she was forced to give up her practice and had to move back to her hometown, where she established a clinic in a rented hotel for $1 a month.

From 1935 to 1942, she operated a cancer clinic. Family members were her staff. By then she had received much publicity for her cancer work.

Each day with a written prescription from their doctors, she would treat many people. Many patients attested to the value of Essiac.

People even filed petitions to get a bill passed recognizing Essiac through the legislature but they failed.

René always believed powerful and influential people were working against her efforts. For years, the medical establishment did not stop her from administering Essiac to cancer patients, because she did not charge anything, although she did accept donations.

Finally, in 1941, the government forced her to close her clinic and she gave up the fight. She then returned home and lived in seclusion. Then in 1977 due to publicity about Essiac, René came out of seclusion. When she was almost ninety she entrusted the secret Essiac formula to the then Lieutenant Governor and a year before her death gave the formula to a Toronto-based company.

Essiac has never been accepted by the medical establishment. However, it is still in wide use, thanks to her sharing the formula with others.

Scientists have evaluated the ingredients of Essiac and concluded that Sheep Sorrel supports the endocrine system. Burdock root eliminates free radicals and purifies the blood. Slippery elm affects the inflammatory balance, and Turkish rhubarb root helps the body eliminate waste and toxins.

Essiac did not "cure" cancer in everyone and René Caisse never claimed it was a cancer "cure".

When the Canadian government shut her clinic down, she went to the United States, where she worked from 1959 to 1967 with a Dr. Charles Brusch. They became partners and co-developers of an improved formula of Essiac.

Dr. Brusch discovered that four additional herbs improved Essiac's effectiveness. After Caisse's death, Dr. Brusch grew impressed with the Paulhus family's (www.bulk-essiac-tea.com) commitment to referring others to Essiac and passed the eight-herb formula to them with the condition that they make Essiac available to everyone at a fair price-- that no one would be denied access to Essiac because of his/her financial situation.

BEWARE! Many companies sell Essiac in the tincture form (in alcohol) or in gelatin capsules, and neither form is true Essiac. True Essiac is a decoction, meaning not an infusion. (An infusion is when you put a tea bag in a cup of hot water. Infusion extracts vitamins and volatile oils.) A decoction extracts the minerals by boiling the ingredients for ten minutes and then allowing the mixture to steep for hours.

In addition, many manufacturers substitute Yellow Dock herb (less effective) for Sheep Sorrel, because Sheep Sorrel is very expensive. The four additional herbs that Dr. Brusch and René Caisse added are:

<u>Blessed Thistle</u> Used in the medieval times to fight the plague, blessed thistle is also used to cleanse the liver, especially when the liver disease is brought on by alcoholism. It contains B-complex vitamins, iron, calcium and manganese.

<u>Red Clover</u> Used as a cancer poultice, specifically skin cancer

<u>Kelp</u> Rich in iodine and alkali

<u>Watercress</u> Contains significant amounts of iron, calcium, iodine and folic acid. Watercress also contains anti-angiogenic cancer-suppressing inhibitors. (Anti-angiogenic inhibitors are used to inhibit solid cancer from growing its own blood vessels.)

Here is the Paulhus' web site: www.bulk-essiac-tea.com

I am impressed with their honesty and dedication to provide their customers with a quality product, along with the fact that Dr. Brusch entrusted them with the eight-herb formula under the condition that they would provide everyone Essiac at a fair price.

The Hoxsey Therapy

On his deathbed, Harry Hoxsey's father passed this cancer treatment formula on to him with the understanding that Harry would turn no one away because of finances.

Harry Hoxsey began "curing" cancer in the 1920s, just around the time the American Medical Association (AMA) began controlling the medical industry.

When the AMA learned of his treatment, Morris Fishburn the head of the AMA, went after Hoxsey through the court system; but Hoxsey fought back. To avoid being arrested for practicing medicine, Harry opened a clinic in Dallas, which was staffed by professional doctors and nurses.

When the medical industry saw that he was gaining recognition and "cutting into their profits," they ganged up on him, "unleashing" the AMA, FDA and NCI (National Cancer Institute) on him. They constantly kept trying to put him out of business through the court system. Finally (in 1960), after the government banned the sale of Hoxsey's formula, Hoxsey moved his clinic to Tijuana, Mexico. In 1974, Harry Hoxsey died of prostate cancer. According to sources, his treatment didn't help him.

To this day, Hoxsey's clinic is still successfully operating, and there is a film entitled, "*When Healing Becomes a Crime*," which is narrated by Max Gail, of *Barney Miller* TV fame. The movie is on youTube. Here is the Hoxsey formula (ten ingredients) with a breakdown of chemical compounds:

1. Licorice Root

Licorice root contains several nitrogen-based chemical compounds, which demonstrate in studies to be anti-tumor and anti-microbial.

2. Red Clover

Red clover, a "green manure crop," adds nutrients (including nitrogen) and other organic matter to the soil. It is grown and plowed under in organic gardening to enrich the soil. Red clover does not contain alkaloids but is still nitrogen-rich.

3. Burdock Root

In the Thistle Family, Burdock root is considered in folk medicine to be a blood-purifying agent. It is used in traditional Chinese medicine.

4. Stillingia Root

American Indians used this root to treat syphilis and other ailments.

5. Oregon Grape

Of all the ingredients, this by far contains the most alkaloids. Oregon grape is not related to grapes you find in the grocery store. Oregon Grape is an evergreen shrub related to barberry.

This shrub contains the potent anti-microbial alkaloid berberine,. I found a total of thirteen alkaloids in Oregon grape. Oregon Grape is in the "top ten list" of plants containing the most alkaloids.

6. Pokeweed

Pokeweed is native to America. According to Wikipedia, all parts of the pokeweed are toxic unless properly prepared. Pokeweed contains at least ten alkaloids, and is one of the top ten medicinal plants containing the most alkaloids.

DID YOU KNOW?

The founders wrote the US Constitution in pokeweed berry ink. Native American Indians used the juice from the pokeweed berry to decorate their horses. Many Civil war letters were written using pokeweed berry ink.

7. Cascara

The Pacific Northwest Indians use the dried, aged bark of the cascara buckthorn as a laxative. Spanish explorers, who observed its effect, called it "Sacred Bark."

Still used today, Cascara bark makes up 20 percent of the laxative market. Studies have shown that one chemical compound (emodin) in Cascara has anti-cancer effects.

My sources did not list any alkaloids in cascara buckthorn.

DID YOU KNOW?

Cascara was widely used in over-the-counter laxative products until May 9, 2002, when the FDA banned the use of cascara and aloe as laxative ingredients in over-the-counter laxatives.

8. Glossy Buckthorn

The bark from this buckthorn is also used as a laxative. No alkaloids were found.

9. Prickly Ash

The bark from the Prickly Ash was used for toothaches, colic and rheumatism. There are at least nine alkaloids present in Prickly Ash.

10. Potassium Iodine (KI)

I have no idea as to the Hoxsey formula's source for iodine, but kelp is rich in potassium iodine.

AUTHOR'S COMMENTS

I felt I had to put this brave man's story in this book.

He was labeled a "quack" by the medical establishment, but he was a hero who fought an expensive legal battle against the medical establishment just to "do the right thing."

His clinic is still open in Mexico. For more information, visit their web site:

www.cancure.org/hoxsey_clinic.htm

Bloodroot

Medicinally used by Native American Indians, bloodroot contains some of the most potent anti-microbial alkaloids in the plant kingdom. A flowering perennial, it is native to eastern North America, from Nova Scotia, Canada all the way down to Florida. It grows well in moist to dry woods, thickets and flood plains.

Bloodroot stores red toxic sap in orange colored rhizomes (roots). The bloodroot plant contains alkaloids, but its rhizome contains some of the most potent and powerful alkaloids known to man:

Berberine ($C_{20}H_{18}NO_4$)

Used in traditional medicine, Berberine has been shown to be effective against fungal infections, Candida, yeast, parasites, and bacteria. Bloodroot's root and rhizome contain 9+ alkaloids, including berberine.

In studies, Berberine has suppressed the growth of tumor cells, including breast cancer, leukemia, melanoma, and pancreatic cancer.

Berberine studies have shown that it has potential for the inhibition and prevention of Alzheimer's. Other plants that contain Berberine are Oregon grape root and Poppyseeds.

Sanguinarine ($C_{20}H_{14}NO_4$)

Of all the alkaloids in the Bloodroot's rhizomes, Sanguinarine is the most prevalent and abundant. In studies, this alkaloid caused apoptosis (programmed cell death) in human cancer cells.

Of course, the FDA warns that bloodroot is ineffective and dangerous as a cancer treatment.

Indian Black Salve

Several companies market bloodroot in a paste or salve. Sellers cannot state that Indian Black Salve is a cancer treatment for fear of prosecution by the FDA.

DID YOU KNOW?

Ants spread Bloodroot seeds, which is called myrmecochory. According to Wikipedia:

> "The seeds have a fleshy organ called an elaiosome that attracts ants. The ants take the seeds to their nest where they eat the elaiosomes and put the seeds in their nest debris, where they are protected until they germinate."

AUTHOR'S COMMENTS

WARNING: Black Salve (bloodroot) is a powerful antimicrobial protocol. Just like the nicotine patch (60+alkaloids), large doses of bloodroot's alkaloids can be toxic and cause death.

If you decide to use bloodroot, follow directions carefully. Buy from a reliable and trustworthy source. My source (not permitted to publish it) uses the <u>correct</u> formula: 25% galangal (ginger root), 25% bloodroot and 50% zinc.

This protocol is potent because you are ingesting the root not extracting the alkaloids.

The Truth about Cinnamon

What we know as cinnamon spice comes from the bark of Cinnamomum trees, which are in the Laurel family (Lauraceae).

According to Wikipedia, a 2007 study at the National Institute of Health showed benefits of cinnamon in the diet of Diabetes type 2 patients. The study claimed cinnamon improved glucose and lipids in people with type 2 Diabetes.

Many medical studies have been done on cinnamon. Some of the compounds studied are:

Eugenol ($C_{10}H_{12}O_2$)

Eugenol is a phenol. According to one study, eugenol extracted from the leaves of the cinnamon tree had anti-viral properties.

Another study claimed eugenol killed human colon cancer cells.

Cinnzeylanine ($C_{22}H_{32}O_7$)

One study showed this compound exhibited anti-viral activity.

Cinnamaldehyde (C_9H_8O)

This chemical compound is the most studied compound in cinnamon. As you can see by its formula, cinnamaldehyde is definitely <u>not</u> an alkaloid. It is a phenol, because cinnamaldehyde gives cinnamon its flavor and aroma. Cinnamaldehyde is described in Wikipedia as:

> "a pale, <u>yellow</u> liquid which occurs naturally in the bark of cinnamon trees."

Wikipedia states that 50% of the essential oil derived from cinnamon bark is cinnamaldehyde.

One study documented cinnamaldehyde's anti-melanoma activity.

What's even more interesting, an Israeli university applied for a patent on a cinnamaldehyde extract they discovered/studied. Their study showed their extract inhibited Alzheimer's disease in laboratory mice.

I am always in seach of the truth. I did not believe the aforementioned cancer studies' findings. I believed there were at least one or more alkaloids involved, but I could not find scientific evidence to prove it. Determined to find the answer, I didn't give up searching for the truth.

I started my search for the mysterious alkaloid(s) by investigating the Lauraceae family, knowing that family members have alkaloids in common. Trees in this family are known for their alkaloids in their bark and roots. Lauraceae alkaloids are classified as Isoquinoline alkaloids. There are several alkaloids classified as Isoquinolines, but one in particular caught my eye:

Berberine ($C_{20}H_{18}NO_4^+$)

Wikipedia describes this alkaloid as:

> "Strongly yellow colored and possesses anti-inflammatory, anti-tumor, and anti-diabetic activities"

This anti-cancer and anti-diabetic activity sounds just like Wikipedia's description of cinnamaldehyde:

> "A pale, yellow liquid, which occurs naturally in the bark of cinnamon trees"

Do you think berberine is the mystery alkaloid in cinnamon? Maybe the following cinnamon facts will convince you it is:

- Studies show cinnamon has anti-fungal properties and Candida cannot live in a cinnamon environment.
- Cinnamon reduces the proliferation of leukemia and lymphoma cells.
- Cinnamon inhibits bacteria from growing.
- Cinnamon kills bacteria in the mouth.

AUTHOR'S COMMENTS

I think these scientists are "barking" up the wrong tree when they claim eugenol, cinnamaldehyde and/or cinnzeylanine are responsible for the anti-cancer activity. These phytochemicals are not alkaloids.

Since Cinnamon's family members contain berberine in the bark, berberine must be "the missing link." What do you think?

DID YOU KNOW?

You can get the full benefits of cinnamon plus the taste of "gourmet" coffee by adding cinnamon to your coffee grounds before brewing.

Recently, a 104-year-old man was on the news. When asked what his secret to longevity was, he replied, "cinnamon and garlic."

Cinnamon Protocol

Like the baking soda and maple syrup protocol, this would be an excellent way to use honey as the "carrier" to get the cinnamon inside the cancer cell to kill the mycoplasma.

Use a ratio of one teaspoon of cinnamon to two teaspoons honey.

Dosage: Once a day

AUTHOR'S COMMENTS

Use raw honey.

Vietnamese cinnamon is the best and highest quality.

Since this is a non-alkalizing protocol, it can be used with the baking soda protocol.

Turmeric

Turmeric and ginger are in the same family, Zingiberaceae. Turmeric is native to tropical south Asia and needs to live in a temperature between 68 and 86 degrees. It needs a considerable amount of rainfall to survive.

The part of both turmeric and ginger that are used medicinally is their rhizomes. Wikipedia's description of rhizomes is:

> "Stems of a plant that are usually found underground"

When I think of rhizomes, I think of an iris, which has roots that grow both in the ground and on the surface.

Turmeric is famous for the spice curcumin. Of all the spices, curcumin has been the most scientifically researched and written about in health food articles.

Curcumin ($C_{21}H_{20}O_6$)

Curcumin has been an ingredient in curry powders for over 2500 years.

Research studies show compounds in turmeric have anti-fungal and anti-bacterial properties, but Wikipedia emphatically states it is not curcumin, a phenol. (Phenols are responsible for aroma.)

Other studies have shown that both turmeric and ginger shrink tumors. A daily dose of curcumin (2 grams) was found to provide pain relief equivalent to ibuprofen for the pain associated with osteoarthritis. According to Dr. Keith Scott, the author of *Medicinal Spices*, curcumin:

- Destroys cancer cells by stimulating apoptosis
- Inhibits formation of abnormal blood vessels (angiogenesis) for tumor growth
- Exhibits properties that help prevent Alzheimer's and Parkinson's diseases

Because of its anti-cancer properties, I suspect turmeric contains a mystery alkaloid–maybe more. Wikipedia's description of curcumin:

> "A distinctly earthy, slightly <u>bitter</u>, slightly <u>hot peppery</u> flavor and a <u>mustard</u> smell"

Notice the words "bitter," "mustard" and "hot peppery." This "reeks" of both an alkaloid (bitter/hot peppery) and a glucosinolate (mustard contains glucosinolates) being present.

Ginger

In China, tea brewed from ginger is a medicinal for colds. Ginger ale is used as a stomach settler.

In India, ginger paste is applied to the temples to relieve headaches. It is also used in India to treat colds.

In the Philippines, ginger is used as a throat lozenge to relieve sore throats.

FYI: Ginger can cause heartburn, bloating, gas, belching and nausea.

Capsaicin ($C_{18}H_{27}NO_3$)

Experts state this alkaloid is present in the ginger <u>plant</u> but not in the rhizome. (This alkaloid is responsible for the chili pepper's "hot" taste.)

NOTE: This might be the alkaloid responsible for the hot peppery taste of turmeric and ginger rhizomes.

Curcumin ($C_{21}H_{20}O_6$)

Curcumin is present in ginger rhizome.

AUTHOR'S COMMENTS

As of this writing, I finally found proof that nitrogen is present in ginger rhizome.

There are definitely more yet-to-be-discovered alkaloids present in both ginger and turmeric rhizomes.

Wikipedia states that ginger has been shown to be active against e-Coli, which proves that there are alkaloids working in the background.

Someday, scientific studies will discover the "mystery" alkaloids in both turmeric and ginger rhizomes.

Ginger/Turmeric Protocol

This is exactly the same protocol ratio as the cinnamon protocol.

Use a ratio of one teaspoon of ginger or turmeric to two teaspoons honey.

Note: For more potency, use fresh grated ginger root

Dosage: Once a day

Variation: Alternate ginger and turmeric

AUTHOR'S COMMENTS

Use raw honey.

Since this is a non-alkalizing protocol, it can be used with the baking soda protocol.

Castor Oil

In the middle ages, castor oil was referred to as "The Palm of Christ," meaning that castor oil packs applied to an injury or wound had the healing effect of Jesus.

This is a remarkable medicinal plant. Ingesting the "raw" seed, however, is lethal.

In 2007 *The Guiness Book of World Records* listed it as the most poisonous plant in the world.

Ricin ($C_{21}H_{16}FN_4OS$)

This chemical compound is what makes the raw castorbean the most poisonous plant in the world. Just ingesting four raw beans is enough to kill an adult.

Symptoms of poisoning are a burning sensation in the mouth and throat, abdominal pain, vomiting, nausea, bloody diarrhea, hypoventilation and seizures, which persist for up to a week. If victims have not died after a week, they recover.

DID YOU KNOW?

In 1978, a Bulgarian dissident by the name of George Markov was assassinated by being stabbed with the point of an umbrella while waiting at a bus stop in London. After his death, a perforated metallic pellet was found embedded in his leg. The pellet contained the deadly toxin ricin. It is suspected that his criticism of communism caused the Bulgarian government to silence him through the KGB.

Fortunately, this toxic substance is extracted in the manufacturing process of castor oil. Manufacturers of castor oil have perfected the system of extracting the deadly poison.

Not only is castor oil super anti-microbial, the following three chemical compounds are responsible for castor oil's effectiveness in the healing process when applied in "heated" topical packs to the abdomen or to the site of a wound or injury:

Albumin ($C_{23}H_{193}N_{35}O_{37}$)

Albumin protein makes up 60 percent of the human blood plasma proteins. These proteins regulate blood volume and act as "taxi cabs," meaning they are carriers of molecules such as nutrients, minerals, and vitamins.

Edestin ($C_{32}H_{39}NO_2$)

This important amino acid is also in hemp seed. Edestin (also spelled Edestine) is a globulin amino acid.

FYI: The definition of globulin: <u>One</u> of the <u>three</u> types of proteins (globulin, albumin and fibrinogen) found in serum, i.e., blood plasma.

The human body uses globulins as building blocks to manufacture many enzymes, hemoglobin, antibodies, DNA and hormones.

Squalene ($C_{30}H_{50}$)

In the body, squalene is the precursor for the manufacturing of cholesterol, steroidal hormones and Vitamin D.

DID YOU KNOW?

Scientists believe squalene has something to do with sharks' longevity and immunity to cancer. Sharks caught and killed for the squalene in their livers, are used to make health supplements.

Military personnel in the 1991 Persian Gulf War, who have squalene antibodies in their bodies, claim that squalene was present in Anthrax vaccinations they received before deployment to Iraq.

A researcher/doctor at Tulane University found that deployed Persian Gulf War Syndrome patients (95 percent) had squalene antibodies present in their bodies. The government was accused of using squalene as an adjuvant in the vaccinations administered to these particular soldiers. Further the only soldiers deployed to Iraq who <u>did not</u> receive the Anthrax vaccine were the French. Was it a coincidence that not one French soldier had squalene antibodies in their bloodstream?

Vaccination Adjuvant

An adjuvant is in vaccinations to aid in the immune response to help an antigen attain the desired immune response.

Wikipedia's definition of an adjuvant:

> "An immunologic adjuvant is defined as any substance that acts to accelerate, prolong or enhance antigen-specific immune responses when used in conjunction with specific vaccine antigens."

In the US, manufacturers of vaccines use Alum (aluminum hydroxide) as an adjuvant. No, your eyes are not deceiving you. They use a form of aluminum in flu shots.

In Europe MF59 is used, which is squalene.

Author's Comments

The government refused to take responsibility for the damage done to the Iraq soldiers who received the Anthrax vaccine. I can only imagine what has happened to those soldiers whose own immune systems destroyed what squalene they had left in their bodies. Even if they ingest squalene, the immune system antibodies would forever identify squalene as a foreign invader and destroy it.

Adjuvants are referred to as *"dirty little secrets"* in the scientific community.

Benefits of Castor Oil

According to Dr. William A. McGarey, the author of the book, *The Oil that Heals*, some benefits Edgar Cayce mentioned in his teachings regarding castor oil are:

- Increases elimination
- Stimulates the liver
- Dissolves and removes lesions
- Stimulates the gall bladder
- Reduces inflammation
- Dissolves gallstones
- Stimulates organs and glands
- Coordinates liver-kidney function

One of Edgar Cayce's remedies for many illnesses was a topical pack soaked in castor oil, placed on the belly and stimulated by the heat of an electrical heating pad. The heat of the heating pad helped the body absorb the healing compounds and alkaloids. (A large percentage of the immune system is located in the digestive tract.)

Amazing speedy healings of lesions, injuries and wounds have been reported.

Ear Infections

By placing drops of castor oil in a child's infected ears has cleared up an infection and eliminated the need for drainage tubes.

Toenail Fungus

Plagued for years with toenail fungus, I tried everything. Nothing worked, until I tried gauze soaked in castor oil wrapped around my infected toenail. I also lifted up the nail and applied castor oil to the nail bed (underneath the nail) with a Q-Tip. Within ONE day, the toenail went from brownish in color to jet black. Three days later (after repeated application of castor oil), the toenail fell off (on its own) and the fungus never returned. The toenail grew back.

Author's Comments

The list goes on and on about the wonderful healing effects and anti-microbial potency of castor oil.

My search for the truth did not uncover any alkaloids in the castor bean; however, I am positive there are yet-to-be-discovered alkaloids present. It is just a matter of time.

Castor Oil Protocol

You will need:

- Castor oil
- Flannel cloth
- Electric heating pad
- Plastic sheeting (saran wrap)
- Bath towel

Step One

Fold flannel cloth (at least four times) to be able to cover area of treatment. (10 x 14 inches finished size)

Step Two

Pour castor oil onto cloth, saturating it but not to the point of dripping.

Step Three

Place saturated cloth on belly or area of treatment. Place plastic sheeting over saturated cloth and then heating pad on top of that

Step Four

Turn heating pad on low and slowly turn up heat. The objective is to heat the area so the body will absorb the castor oil, but not burn the patient.

Step Five

When heat is set high enough where the patient is still comfortable, place bath towel over heating pad to keep heat from escaping. Folded bath towel should cover entire trunk of patient. One to one-and-a-half hours is the normal treatment time.

Author's Comments

Dr. McGaray recommends taking a teaspoonful of olive oil after treatment to stimulate the liver.

Recommended number of treatments per week: Three to seven

Note: The cloth pack is reusable. If need be, add more castor oil to pack. When not in use, keep in plastic bag in refrigerator. Discard if rancid.

Source: *The Oil that Heals* by William A. McGaray, MD

Venus Flytrap

The Venue Flytrap is a carnivorous plant whose source of food can range from beetles to spiders to arthropods. (An arthropod is an insect with an external skeleton.) Its preferred diet, however, consists of beetles, spiders, ants and grasshoppers. Very seldom can it catch flying insects. How the plant traps its victim is as follows:

When a potential dinner crawls along its leaves and comes in contact with a "hair", the trap closes only when another hair is touched (within twenty seconds of the first encounter). This is to ensure against wasting energy.

Only then, will the leaf close, trapping the victim inside. The prey's movement only causes the leaf to close even tighter, forming a stomach where digestion can begin. Digestion starts by the release of plumbagin and enzymes. Wikipedia describes plumbagin ($C_{11}H_8O_3$) as a toxin. Digestion takes around ten days at which time the prey is reduced to a husk of chitin. The trap then reopens and is ready for its next meal.

Carnivora, which is made from the pure phytonutrients of the Venus Flytrap (Dionaea muscipula) was first developed in Germany in the late 1970s by the German physician Dr. Helmut Keller, who discovered its immune-supporting properties.

It is now manufactured in America under the name Carnivora, and information regarding Carnivora can be found on Carnivora Research, Inc.'s web site: www.carnivora.com.

Their web site lists seventeen of Carnivora's chemical compounds, several of which are essential and non-essential amino acids (eight). One phytochemical in particular caught my eye:

Lipopolysaccharide

Wikipedia's definition of lipopolysaccharides is:

> "..........Large molecules of a lipid and a polysaccharide.........they are found in the outer membrane of Gram-negative bacteria and act as endotoxins and induce a strong immune response in animals."

Did you notice that lipopolysaccharides are endotoxins that induce immune response? Mycoplasmas are Gram-negative bacteria and their outer membrane consists of lipopolysaccharides!

In my opinion, a lipopolysaccharide is to the immune system as a drop of blood is to a shark, which triggers a feeding frenzy!

Another phytochemical found in Carnivora is Hydroplumbagin, which the maker of Carnivora describes as "immune modulation/stimulation." Wikipedia describes hydro as "fluid" and Plumbagin ($C_{11}H_8O_3$) as "a toxin."

In studies Carnivora has been found to <u>stimulate</u> the immune system to kill the AIDS virus. (This makes sense because the membrane of the AIDS virus (mycoplasma) is made up of lipopolysaccharides-- endotoxins.)

AUTHOR'S COMMENTS

I would not hesitate to "bet the ranch" that the lipopolysaccharide(s) in Carnivora are the phytochemicals, which stimulate an immune response.

The makers of Carnivora proclaim that after taking only three capsules of Carnivora, within three hours the immune system's cells are up and running and doing what they are programmed to do.

For more information, visit their web site:

www.carnivora.com

A Medicinal Garden

Someday, we may have no other choice but to take responsibility for our own health and heal ourselves, just as our ancestors did.

The following are medicinal plants you can grow yourself–many of them considered invasive weeds.

#1 Marigold

Go to page 148 for chapter on Marigolds.

#2 Vinca Minor

This plant is in the top five medicinal plants. It has at least 50 documented alkaloids. For more information, it is listed in Plant-Based Protocols. See Vinca Minor chapter and protocol, page 144.

#3 Dandelions

Dandelions are in the Asteraceae family. Used in Europe, North America and China, this plant is an herbal remedy, used to treat bile and liver problems and infections. Flowers are used to make dandelion wine, greens are used in salads and the 3-4 year old root is used to make coffee.

<u>Prunasin</u> ($C_{14}H_{17}NO_6$) is a cyanogenic glycoside found in the root of the dandelion. This is very important, because cyanogenic glycosides kill pathogens, especially mycoplasmas. (Cyanogenic glycosides are explained in the "Defending" section.)

<u>Dandelion Coffee</u> - Mature roots are dried, roasted, and then ground up to make coffee. Dandelion coffee has a bitter taste, probably because of nitrogen in the root. (Plants put nitrogen in their roots to protect themselves from microorganisms in the soil.)

<u>Nitrogen</u> - The green leaves and stems of the plant are an excellent source of nitrogen.

#4 Yarrow

This is another flowering plant in the amazing Asteraceae family. Its genus name, Achillea millefolium is derived from the mythical Greek character Achilles, who carried yarrow with him to treat soldiers' wounds. Yarrow poultice is known to staunch (stop) the flow of blood from wounds.

Typically, plants in the same family have phytochemicals in common, especially nitrogen-based chemical compounds. There are at least seven documented alkaloids and nitrogen-based phytochemicals found in the plant:

Yarrow is sweet with a slightly bitter taste (alkaloids). Yarrow was very popular as a food in the 17th century. The young leaves were cooked like spinach and added to soups. Today, dried leaves are used as an herb in cooking. According to Wikipedia:

> "The dark blue essential oil extracted by steam distillation of the flowers is generally used as an anti-inflammatory or in chest rubs for colds and influenza."

According to sources, yarrow intensifies the medicinal action of other herbs. Yarrow is associated with the following treatments:

- Pain
- Bleeding
- Gastrointestinal disorders
- Inflammation
- Stomachache

Chinese medicinal practitioners claim yarrow brightens the eyes and promotes intelligence.

Native Americans considered yarrow to be a "life medicine" and chewed it for toothaches and poured an infusion into ears for earaches. Some Native Americans used it to treat head colds. Other Native Americans used the leaves for headaches by inhaling steam.

#5 Burdock

This plant craves nitrogen, which signifies that it is high in nitrogen-based phytochemicals. Another plant that is in the Asteraceae family, Burdock is grown for its root, which is used as a vegetable.

Historically known as a blood purifier, burdock is one of the components of Essiac Tea. A detoxifier of the lymph and the liver, it is a diuretic (promotes urination) and a diaphoretic (promotes perspiration).

Other parts of the plant are used to fight infections, acne, boils, poison ivy and oak, as a tonic and a mild laxative. Traditional Chinese medicine uses burdock seeds for skin conditions and for colds and the flu.

DID YOU KNOW?

In the 1940s, a Swiss inventor by the name of George de Mestral was curious as to how Burdock seeds stuck to his clothes and to his dog's fur. Using a microscope, he observed the "hook" system that the seed used to latch on to passing animals, which aided in the seed's dispersal. Mestral realized that this "hook-type" system could be used to join things together. The result of his invention was Velcro.

#6 Stevia

Stevia is another plant (stevia rebaudiana) in the remarkable family of Asteraceae. This plant is the plant that you hear so much controversy about. Used as a natural sweetener, the FDA has been persecuting manufacturers of Stevia. Here is why:

Studies have shown that stevia kills cancer cells (mycoplasma). This is why pharmaceuticals use the FDA to harass and persecute alternative medicinal competition. Many countries ban stevia. Sellers of stevia cannot promote stevia as a sweetener, only as a dietary supplement.

In the US, it is still legal to grow your own stevia. Stevia grows well in a hydroponic unit and does well in container gardens. Just like its sibling the marigold, stevia need lots of sunlight. The plants are hard to germinate, but purchase live plants from:

www.herabladvantage.com

The Herbal Advantage, Route 3, Box 93, Rogersville MO 65742

www.wellsweep.com

Well Sweep Herb Farm, 205 Mt. Bethel Road, Port Murray, NJ 07895

https://www.richters.com

Richter's Herbs, 357 Highway 47, Goodwood, Ontario LOC-IA0

To learn how to grow your own stevia, buy on Amazon *The Stevia Story* by Donna Gates. Read her article on this web site:

www.stevia.net/growingstevia.htm

For the stevia protocol, visit www.cancertutor.com and look under "Dirt Cheap Protocols."

Avoid stevia products with dextrose. Trader Joe's has a stevia product that is dextrose-free. (Dextrose is a form of glucose.) There is a stevia product called Sweet Leaf.

#7 Other Asteraceae Plants

The following are some other plants in the amazing family that you can grow:

- o   Daisies (relieves headaches, muscle pain and allergy symptoms)
- o   Chrysanthemums (used as an insecticide [Pyrethrum)])
- o   Artichokes (aids digestion and gall bladder function)
- o   Blessed Thistle (cleanses liver)
- o   Sunflowers (#1 on arginine list)

#8 Impatiens (Jewelweed)

This is a very popular annual available in just about every color of the rainbow, except yellow or blue. Used as a topical to prevent a rash from contact with poison ivy, scientific studies have shown once the rash appears, the ointment is useless.

It is used as a topical for bee stings, insect bites and stinging nettle. According to Wikipedia, impatiens taste "bitter" and are slightly toxic. This tells me that there are alkaloids present.

DID YOU KNOW?

One of the phytochemicals in impatiens is an active ingredient in Preparation H.

#9 Plantain

After reading this chapter, you may never put down herbicides on your lawn again.

Plantains are invasive weeds that grow in the spring. They have a broad leaf and are very green. The weed plantain is not to be confused with a type of banana named plantain.

Used as far back as prehistoric times, this plant is an herbal remedy.

According to Wikipedia:

> "The herb is astringent, anti-toxic, antimicrobial, anti-inflammatory, anti-histimine, as well as demulcent, expectorant, styptic, and diuretic."

A poultice of leaves is used for insect bites, poison ivy, rashes, minor sores and boils. As a tea, tincture or syrup and used for coughs and bronchitis, the broad leaf variety can be eaten as salad greens. There are at least six nitrogen-based phytochemicals found in plantain.

Plantains are high in nitrogen and are easier to grow than lettuce. They like water and nitrogen-rich soil. The more nitrogen in the soil, the more the plant will convert nitrogen into nitrogen-based phytochemicals.

#10 Shepherd's Purse

This plant is in the same family (Brassicaceae) as broccoli, cauliflower, mustard, etc. One of the family's characteristics is glucosinolates, which are alkaloids plus sulfur. Shepherd's Purse has three.

Traditional Austrian medicine uses Shepherd Purse internally in teas or in a tincture to treat cardiovascular and gynecologic problems. Externally, they use Shepherd's Purse to treat skin disorders.

#11 Mullein (Verbascum)

This flowering perennial can grow up to 9.8 feet tall. Medicinally, all of the plant, including the flowers, is used. According to Wikipedia:

> "Flowers have been used in the traditional Austrian medicine internally (as tea) or externally (as ointment) for treatment of disorders of the respiratory tract, skin veins, gastrointestinal tract and the locomotive system."

The leaves of this plant stimulate coughing, which clears the lungs. Infused oil can be used for ear infections.

#12 Dock & Sorrel

There are over 200 species of annual and perennial plants in the buckwheat family.

According to Wikipedia:

> "In traditional Austrian medicine Rumex alpinis leaves and roots have been used internally for treatment of viral infections."

In most areas, these plants are a nuisance and considered weeds.

The Rife Machine

Everything has a frequency (vibration), including humans and even microorganisms.

Dr. Royal Rife was one of the most brilliant inventors in medical history, but his invention and contributions to the field of medicine have been suppressed for decades.

Not until recently, has his technology resurfaced to be used for what he originally invented it to be used for--the killing of pathogenic microorganisms.

Not only was Dr. Rife brilliant, but he was also a humanitarian, who was determined to find the cure for disease and cancer. Unfortunately, even though he proved his invention worked, his ideas were so advanced, that the medical establishment rejected them.

In the 1920s, Dr. Rife set out to prove that every organism has its own individual frequency (vibration). During his research, he also discovered that an organism is sensitive to its own specific frequency and could be killed by intensifying this frequency until the organism exploded. (Picture a human voice shattering a glass.)

To kill the microorganisms by frequency, Rife invented what he called a "frequency tube," which is a primitive version of the Rife machine today.

Dr. Rife encountered many obstacles, one of them being that none of the microscopes in the 1920s could view a tiny virus. At that time, it was impossible. (Using white-light microscopes, microorganisms become invisible. Also, if an organism is stained (standard protocol) with a chemical, the chemical kills it. This was of no help to Dr. Rife. He needed to see and experiment on "live" microorganisms.

To prove that his invention worked, not only did he have to see the organism, the organism had to be alive so he could try and kill it. So before he could even prove his "frequency tube" worked, he had to invent a microscope powerful enough to see a "live" virus.

By the 1930s, Dr. Rife had accomplished the impossible! He had built the first virus microscope, which was capable of magnifying objects 60,000 times their normal size.

Amazingly, Rife was the first human being to see a "live" virus. How was this possible–to see a once-invisible organism? Again, organisms are invisible under regular white-light microscopes, but the theory behind Rife's microscope was that each type of microorganism became visible in a unique color of its own when it was exposed to the color frequency that resonated with its own unique vibration.

Using a spectroscope, Dr. Rife painstakingly identified each individual frequency of each known microbe. When this task was completed, he was then ready to prove his "frequency tube" worked.

By slowly rotating the crystal prisms and focusing light on the organism under his virus microscope, Dr. Rife was able to see "live" microorganisms invading human cells!

Then, with the organisms in his sights, they became "sitting ducks." Using his frequency tube, he "blasted" the organisms with their own intensified frequency, instantly exploding and killing them.

His theory and invention worked! He had killed microorganisms that caused disease and cancer. (This also proves that cancer and disease are infections!)

Before trying his invention on humans, he experimented on lab animals. Over and over again, he would infect the same lab animals with cancer and get them well.

Not until then was he ready to try his invention on humans. Amazingly, the only cancer patients available were 20 stage four cancer patients who had been given no chance of recovery. Amazingly, he got <u>every</u> single one of them well.

This resulted in "negative" attention from the pharmaceutical industry and the AMA.

Unfortunately, life was not kind to Dr. Rife. Shortly thereafter, all of his equipment and documentation were destroyed from outside forces.

Then, sadly, after many years of persecution and abuse, Dr. Rife's life was destroyed, too. Suffering from alcoholism, he mysteriously died in 1971. (Rumors suggest he was poisoned.)

AUTHOR'S COMMENTS

Even Dr. Rife in the 1920s had something to say about the correlation between an "unbalanced" cell and disease. The following Dr. Rife quote appears in *The Cancer Cure That Worked* written by Barry Lynes:

> "In reality, it is not the bacteria themselves that produce the disease, but the chemical constituents of these microorganisms enacting upon the unbalanced cell metabolism of the human

body that in actuality produce the disease. We also believe if the metabolism of the human body is perfectly balanced or poised, it is susceptible to no disease."

The Zapper

Dr. Hulda Clark was a well-known cancer researcher who focused on human diseases, especially cancer. She discovered many ways to rid the body of pathogens, i.e., parasites, bacteria, viruses and fungus. She also focused on environmental factors, which included heavy metals, solvents and even radioactivity.

Her most important invention was what she named "the Zapper". Zapping "electrocutes" pathogens. Some people use the term "vitalizes the blood," which means the Zapper vitalizes the pathogen's environment.

Dr. Clark did not recommend pregnant women or people on pacemakers to use a Zapper, because no research has been done.

Dr. Clark has written seven books, five concerning cancer. In them, she shares her methods, results and conclusions to give the reader a self-help approach to getting well.

She was a great humanitarian, who was always under attack by the medical establishment and the government for her research and contributions to alternative medicine. Sadly, Dr. Clark passed away on September 3, 2009.

Today's typical Zapper consists of a plastic case, which is about 2"x4"x1.3" deep. The Zapper runs on a 9-volt battery, which is inside the case. The Zapper is placed and held against the skin with some sort of bandage. (I use an old sock with both ends open so I can wear it on my arm. Inside the sock, the Zapper is snugly pressed against the skin.) When switched on, the Zapper emits 30 KHz (30,000 cycles per second--Dr. Hulda Clark determined that this was the ideal charge). The Zapper's pulses are not painful nor are they uncomfortable.

UPDATE - The Best Zapper

There are many Zapper sellers on the Internet, but I believe the best and most effective one is "The Best Zapper."

www.bestzapper.com

Silver (Ag)

Documentation of silver used for anti-microbial purposes can be traced back to the Phoneticians (1550 to 300 BC), who stored water, wine, and vinegar in silver bottles to prevent spoiling. Even Hippocrates (480 to 370 BC), who is the "Father of Western Medicine," wrote of its healing and anti-disease properties.

It was also common for our ancestors to put silver bars in their wells, drink out of silver chalices, or put silver coins in water pitchers to kill microorganisms.

Silver is a metallic element, which has the highest electrical conductivity of all the elements (even more than copper [Cu] which is used in electrical wiring).

ANTI-MICROBIAL

Today, there are three types of silver treatments available: Ionic Silver, Colloidal Silver, and Mild Silver Protein.

Ionic Silver (Ag^+)

Of the three treatments, this is the most <u>ineffective</u> and potentially the most harmful type of silver to use. Here is why:

It is all about chemistry. Ionic silver is missing a negative electron (see above formula), which makes ionic silver positive ($^+$). This also makes it highly receptive to "hooking up" with an opposite (negatively charged) ion ($^-$). (Opposites attract.)

After ingestion, ionic silver enters the stomach, where it immediately latches onto an oppositely charged ion--usually chloride (Cl$^-$). (Notice the negative sign.). According to Wikipedia, chloride is a "chemical that the body needs for metabolism (the process of turning food into energy). Chloride also helps keep the body's acid/base balance." (FYI: Kidneys control chloride levels in the blood.)

When chloride and silver (ions) form, they become harmless salts, which are eliminated through excretion. There are no anti-microbial properties in silver chloride (ClAg).

In summary, ionic silver is worthless for killing microorganisms on the "inside." However, as a topical dressing or for treating a wound, it can be effective. Many sellers of ionic silver know that buyers are not "savvy" as to ionic silver's internal ineffectiveness against pathogens. Beware of ionic silver labels such as "Monaionic silver," "Silver hydrosol," and "Covalent silver." These are all ionic silver. FYI: There is also no such thing as ionic silver particles.

ARGYRIA

According to an article on www.purestcolloids.com, the man renowned as "The Blue Man" was a "disinformation" campaign paid for by a pharmaceutical company to scare the public into thinking colloidal silver causes Argyria. On the contrary, the true story goes that he unknowingly made a homemade brew of ionic silver and salt (silver chloride) and applied it to his skin. Then he used a tanning bed to "fix" the silver in his body, and the rest is history. You can read the full story by Googling the following phrase:

"By now everyone has seen the story about Paul Karason"

Again, Argyria results from over-ingesting <u>large-sized</u> particles of silver and/or ionic silver. Signs of this condition are blue or bluish-gray skin. Reliable, <u>unbiased</u> sources state Argyria is caused by ionic silver.

One source, www.purestcolloids.com, in an article entitled *The Truth about Ionic Silver*, states the following:

"Ingestion of high concentrated forms of ionic silver (100 ppm and above) may cause Argyria, a permanent discoloration of the skin."

Colloidal Silver (Ag)

This is the "over-the-counter" silver product of choice for killing cancer or disease-causing organisms. However, all colloidal silver products are not created equal.

Effective colloidal silver's particles are <u>very tiny</u> and are measured in nanometers. Unlike ionic silver, colloidal silver does not "combine" with negative or positively charged ions or molecules in the body. Colloidal silver is metallic.

ANTI-MICROBIAL EFFECTS

Colloidal silver is lethal to microorganisms, such as mycoplasma. When silver comes into contact with a pathogen, such as mycoplasma, it deactivates its metabolic enzymes and destroys the outer cell membrane, which kills the mycoplasma. According to sources, mycoplasma has not been able to adapt or avoid the silver's lethal effect on its membrane. The same effect applies to bacteria and fungus.

CONCLUSION

Before buying a colloidal silver product, Google the following key word phrase:

"How to tell if a product is mostly ionic silver"

This is an article, which rates the current colloidal silver and ionic silver products on the market.

The rule of thumb is a solution that has a high percentage of colloidal silver and a very low percentage of ionic silver.

From what I have learned, it is near impossible to obtain a pure (100%) solution of colloidal silver. Ionic silver will always be present (a by-product) in the production of colloidal silver.

Mild Silver Protein

On the advice of Dr. Harold Clark who I had talked to at the Canadian mycoplasma conference in 2005, when I returned home I immediately started calling alternative doctors around the country looking for an IV treatment of tetracycline, which was the only known treatment for a mycoplasma infection at that time.

I live in St. Louis, Missouri, which is in the middle of the country, so I could go anywhere, but I was disappointed. Phone call after phone call, I was unsuccessful. I could find no alternative doctor who would administer a tetracycline IV. Disheartened, I found myself at the end of a long list of possible alternative doctors, and there was only one left within one day's driving distance. He was located in Birmingham, Alabama.

When I called him, he answered the phone himself. I asked him about a tetracycline treatment and he said, "I've got another treatment. I've cured AIDS, chronic fatigue, and Diabetes!"

The treatment was an IV of mild silver protein (MSP) which is nano-size colloidal silver suspended in a matrix of protein. From reading articles about mild silver protein, MSP is not the same as plain colloidal silver. Mild silver protein is very effective against mycoplasma and other pathogenic organisms (fungus, bacteria and especially the Lyme spirochaete) when administered through an IV.

From what this doctor told me, MSP administered through an IV, "interferes with cellular metabolic machinery and structure and kills the pathogen." The doctor also advised that if I had an infection, I would go through the Herxheimer's (kill-off) within two hours of the treatment.

He was right. Within two hours, my body started reacting from the killoff. I had flu-like symptoms (chills and fever). The Herxheimer reaction lasted around three hours.

Amazingly, the next morning (Sunday) when I woke up, I felt like a new person. There was no pain in my joints. I could even get up from the bed unassisted, and I felt wonderful!

Sunday was a day of rest, and Monday I received my second IV of MSP. Since I had no negative reaction to the silver during my first IV treatment, I was allowed to go home after the IV drip was over; but that didn't mean I wouldn't go through more Herxheimer's—that, I experienced on the way home in the car.

Coincidentally, that same week I had an appointment with my doctor in St. Louis. My blood test results came back "negative" for lupus! MSP had killed the mycoplasmas.

AUTHOR'S COMMENTS

Doctors are fearful that the FDA and/or the FBI will raid their offices and shut them down, even though the FDA "grand fathered in" mild silver protein a long time ago.

There are several negative articles on the Internet about mild silver protein. All of the authors refer to mild silver protein as being ingested and the silver particles in mild silver protein are very large in comparison to colloidal silver particles. They claim mild silver protein is inferior.

For more information about mild silver protein, visit my web site

www.lindaemmanuel.com

Sulfur (S)

Sulfur, an element, is essential for all life. Sulfur deficiency leads to cell degeneration and disease or cancer. It also plays a key role in oxygenation and detoxification of the cells. The human body is four percent sulfur but does not store reserves or manufacture sulfur. Sulfur must be ingested--it is an "essential" mineral.

According to sources, in the 1950s the government began mandating farmers use chemical fertilizers. Manmade fertilizers "inhibit" sulfur from working in the body. Because of this, experts theorize that almost every person alive today is "sulfur-deficient."

Further, with heavy coal mining and oil extraction from the soil and the burning of fossil fuels, sulfur is escaping into the air and joins with atmospheric moisture to form sulfuric acid (acid rain). With all of this human activity, less and less sulfur is available to plants, which can only absorb (access) sulfur <u>through the root system</u> (not through the air).

Sulfur is also essential for plant growth, root formation and protection against fungus and insects. Sulfur is added to manmade fertilizers, but this sulfur source is usually a <u>by-product</u> of removing sulfur-containing contaminants from natural gas and petroleum.

Sulfur deficiency is linked to chlorine and fluoride, which inhibit sulfur absorption in the body. Vitamins such as biotin and thiamine contain sulfur.

Glutathione ($C_{10}H_{17}N_3O_6S$)

The following are a few of glutathione's functions in the human body:

- Participates directly with the neutralization of free radicals
- Maintains anti-oxidants (vitamins C and E) in their reduced (active) form
- Used in DNA synthesis and repair
- Participates in enzyme activation
- Used in protein synthesis and amino acid transport
- Is necessary for the cell's uptaking of oxygen (respiration)
- Plays a vital role (function) in iron metabolism
- Regulates the nitric oxide cycle

As you can see, sulfur plays an important role in <u>all</u> functions of the human body, especially the brain.

Sulfur also has other important roles in the body:
- Is largely responsible for the mechanical strength and insolubility of the protein keratin found in the skin and hair
- Disulfide bonds are a major component in holding joints and connective tissue together, making cartilage firm and resilient

Sulfur deficiency can be a factor in joint pain, back pain, sore muscles, headaches, heartburn, cold sores, gray hair, gastrointestinal disorders, and acne, just to name a few.

Studies have shown there is a correlation between low levels of glutathione and cancer/disease.

It is vital to ingest an organic (non-manmade) form of sulfur. It is also important to buy sulfur in a <u>crystalline</u> state. Powdered (capsules) sulfur is not the best choice.

WARNING: Sulfur thins blood. It can also enhance prescriptions. Before taking sulfur supplements, consult your doctor.

DID YOU KNOW?

China is one of the main suppliers of sulfur supplements, which are contaminated by-products of natural gas and petroleum!

The following company has integrity and product quality:

www.h2oairwateramericas.com

Vitamin C Therapy

Vitamin C ($C_6H_8O_6$) is derived from glucose and is a "weak" acidic sugar, meaning that it can easily donate (lose) elements in metabolic processes.

Vitamin C is essential for all animal life. Humans, guinea pigs, monkeys, apes and certain species of bats and birds cannot convert glucose into vitamin C. Because of a genetic mutation, the aforementioned do not manufacture the enzyme L-gulonolactone oxidase, which is the required catalyst to make Vitamin C.

Reptiles and some orders of birds manufacture Vitamin C in their kidneys. Mammals who can make Vitamin C, manufacture it in their livers, where the enzyme is present.

Vitamin C plays a crucial role in enzymatic reactions, especially in the synthesis of collagen (donating electrons, i.e., elements). The presence of Vitamin C is important in wound healing and in preventing bleeding from the capillaries. Most importantly, Vitamin C is an antioxidant, donating electrons to keep iron and copper atoms in their reduced state. (Remember that mycoplasma use copper and iron in their metabolism, which plays a crucial role in why Vitamin C therapy is effective.) Vitamin C also enhances iron absorption.

In summary, humans must have sufficient amounts of Vitamin C, otherwise scurvy will manifest.

Scurvy

Scurvy has plagued man since the beginning of time. It was especially prevalent in the days of sailing vessels when sailors, soldiers and pirates were out to sea for long stretches of time. Their only food supply was salted meat and dried grains, because fruits and vegetables were perishable.

Hippocrates who lived circa 400 BC even described scurvy. Symptoms of scurvy include:

- Malaise and lethargy
- Spongy gums, loose teeth and gum bleeding
- Jaundice and fever
- Wounds not healing

Vitamin C is important to the immune system for healing, especially in the synthesis of collagen.

Author's Comments

Cancer patients have been observed to have low levels of Vitamin C and scurvy symptoms. This is because Vitamin C is in short supply from the drain of infection.

Oral Vitamin C Supplementation

Vitamin C is water soluble and any excess will be eliminated from the body. Oral mega doses of Vitamin C, therefore, are ineffective in the treatment of disease and cancer; and, in fact, "feed" mycoplasmas. (Vitamin C is derived from glucose.)

However, Vitamin C through an IV is an effective treatment against mycoplasmas and I will explain why; but first, I have to explain aerobic cell respiration.

Aerobic Cell Respiration

When the cell is burning molecules to make energy, for example glucose ($C_6H_{12}O_6$), the cell needs a way to get rid of the carbon and the hydrogen elements, which if left unattached in the cell, do great damage to the cell–even causing cell death.

Glucose is a "weak" (electrically charged) acidic molecule, which easily gives up elements (carbon and hydrogen) to a stronger molecule such as oxygen (O_2). Here is the action:

One glucose ($C_6H_{12}O_6$), + six oxygen (O_2) = six carbon dioxides (CO_2) + one water (H_2O)

$$C_6H_{12}O_6 + 6(O_2) = 6(CO_2) + H_2O$$

CO_2 is eliminated through the lungs, and the H_2O is eliminated through the sweat glands and the urinary track.

Hydrogen Peroxide (H_2O_2)

Hydrogen peroxide is a natural byproduct of many metabolic processes.

Within macrophages (immune system cell) enzymes and toxic hydrogen peroxide destroy and digest pathogens.

Hydrogen peroxide is even used by plants as a defense against pathogenic microbes.

Potentially, hydrogen peroxide can damage the cell. Therefore, aerobic life has a natural defensive mechanism--catalase, an enzyme to protect it from the potentially harmful effects of hydrogen peroxide.

Catalase

Catalase is a polypeptide, which consists of over 500 amino acids. It also contains essential iron that allows the enzyme to react upon contact with the hydrogen peroxide.

Catalase converts hydrogen peroxide into water and oxygen. Catalase is recycled and just one catalase enzyme can convert hydrogen peroxide into water and oxygen one million times a second.

Interestingly, "loose" heavy metal ions such as copper and iron inhibit catalase from converting hydrogen peroxide into water and oxygen.

DID YOU KNOW?

A few contact lens-cleaning products contain hydrogen peroxide to kill harmful bacteria. After using this solution, a solution containing catalase breaks down the hydrogen peroxide.

The aerobic Tuberculosis bacterium produces catalase to neutralize hydrogen peroxide, which allows the bacterium to survive inside the macrophage within the lungs.

Mycoplasmas are anaerobic, meaning they do not use oxygen in their metabolism. In fact, in the presence of oxygen, they die. Hydrogen peroxide kills mycoplasmas. In fact, hydrogen peroxide is more lethal to mycoplasmas than bleach.

DID YOU KNOW?

It has been documented that cancer cells uptake glucose 19 times faster than normal cells. The outcome of anaerobic sugar fermentation is lactic acid ($C_3H_6O_3$). (See Cachexia chapter, psge 51.)

Doctors use sugar to detect if cancer cells have metastasized (spread). Before performing a PET scan, the patient is injected with sugar containing radioactive dye. The cancer cells light up like a Christmas tree.

Ironically, doctors tell cancer patients to "fatten up" by eating high sugar food, such as ice cream, which only "feeds" mycoplasmas.

Research has shown that cancer cells, especially, like high fructose corn syrup used to sweeten just about every processed food available in the grocery store. Research has proven that pancreatic cancer cells use high fructose corn sugar to proliferate.

The following is why mega doses of Vitamin C through an IV are effective against mycoplasmas:

Vitamin C IV

Remember that Vitamin C is derived from glucose and that mycoplasmas recognize Vitamin C as a potential meal. Cancer cells (mycoplasmas are inside) uptake sugar 19 times faster than normal cells. Mycoplasmas are hungry for sugar, which enables them to proliferate.

According to researchers who observe the effects of Vitamin C IV therapy, when mega doses of Vitamin C enter the cancer cell (oxygen is not present in the cancer cell), Vitamin C starts interacting with iron and copper that <u>are</u> present in the cancer cell. (There is no catalase enzyme in the cancer cell, because iron and copper inhibit it).

The result of this interaction produces small amounts of hydrogen peroxide. As more and more mega doses of Vitamin C are uptaken by the cancer cell (mycoplasmas), more and more hydrogen peroxide accumulates. Hydrogen peroxide (H_2O_2) is lethal to the pathogenic mycoplasmas and they die!

Author's Comments

It takes mega doses of Vitamin C through an IV to kill mycoplasmas. Amazingly, mycoplasmas make themselves vulnerable by needing iron for metabolic functions.

Many alternative doctors are familiar with Vitamin C therapy and are, therefore, willing to give vitamin C IVs.

Do-It-Yourself Vitamin C

Vitamin C in ascorbic acid form sometimes is destroyed in the digestive process. The following mixture bypasses the digestion process and gets into the bloodstream much easier. You will need:

- Bulk non-GMO sunflower lecithin (suggested source below)
- Bulk ascorbic acid powder (suggested source below)
- Distilled water

Step One

Dissolve three level tablespoons of lecithin in one cup of distilled water in a glass jar or blender.

Shake (or blend) lecithin and distilled water mixture until completely dissolve--no granules are visible.

Step Two

In separate glass bowl, dissolve one level tablespoon of ascorbic acid powder in one-half cup of distilled water.

Step Three

Combine lecithin mixture and ascorbic powder mixture together in ultrasonic cleaner bowl.

> Tip: Before combining mixture in ultrasonic bowl, combine mixtures in a glass jar and screw lid on. Shake.

Pour both mixtures into Ultrasonic bowl (from Walmart) and turn on switch. While mixing, stir with a plastic utensil or straw. Machine will stop every two minutes. Repeat two more times for a total of six minutes, repeatedly stirring mixture.

Step Four

Batch yields around 12 grams of Vitamin C. Mixture will keep at room temperature three to four days. If refrigerated, it will last longer.

John Beard, Father of Enzyme Therapy

John Bead was born on November 2, 1858, in Redding, England. He was born into humble surroundings, where both his father and grandfather worked in local cotton mills.

According to sources, John Beard was ambitious and had a greater goal in life than following in his fathers' footsteps. Eventually, Beard had the opportunity to attend college and finished his PhD from the University of Edinburgh. Then he received an honorary Doctorate of Science from the University of Manchester. He received even further education, specializing in embryology, at the Universities of Würzburg and Freiberg. When he returned to England, he went to work for the Scottish Fishery Board.

Working for the Scottish Fishery Board, Dr. Beard studied sharks, skates and rays. After researching fish for twenty years, he left that position and took the position of assistant lecturer of vertebrate embryology at the University of Edinburgh. This is where he did his embryological studies and developed his theory that there was a similarity between embryonic stem cells and cancer cells, namely trophoblast cells and cancer cells.

Author's Comments

To understand Dr. Beard's theory about enzymes and cancer cells, one must understand concepts about the development of an embryo/fetus.

The Blastocyst

The blastocyst is the structure that is formed <u>around</u> the embryo. The inner cell mass forms the embryo, and the outer cell mass is referred to as trophoblast cell(s), which eventually form the placenta that attaches to the maternal lining of the uterus.

Trophoblast Cells

According to Wikipedia:

> "The trophoblast is a layer of cells forming the outer ring of the blastocyst that combines with the maternal endometrium to form the placenta."

Trophoblast cells secrete enzymes to break down the maternal endometrial cells (lining) to allow penetration and implantation of the blastocyst in the uterine wall.

Author's Comments

The following is the key to understanding WHY John Beard theorized that enzymes were the body's natural defense against caner cells.

Integrin

Trophoblast cells contain Integrin on their outer cell surface, which allows for adhesion of the placenta to the uterine wall.

Many molecules of Integrin span the trophoblast cell membrane. Most importantly, just one molecule of Integrin holds the largest domain of membrane <u>proteins</u> (1,088 amino acids) in the human body. (All these proteins are necessary to guarantee successful attachment of the placenta to the surface of the uterus.)

Cell Adhesion

Cell adhesion is the binding of a cell to a surface or to another cell. Adhesion occurs <u>only</u> from the action of <u>proteins</u>. (Cells in our body are attached to each other with protein.)

Author's Comment

John Beard was actually ahead of his time. In fact, he was a genius. He observed in his embryonic research that trophoblast cells are "parasitic," meaning they are invasive. Not only were they parasitic, they posed a problem if they were not stopped after attaching to the uterine wall.

The problem was that they would continue to grow just like cancer cells, forming a choriocarcinoma (a deadly tumor), threatening the life of both mother and fetus.

The Theory Behind John Beard's Enzyme Therapy

John Beard also noted that by the 56th day of gestation, the fetus' pancreas had developed and was producing trypsin, an enzyme that breaks down protein. He observed that this is when the "parasitic" trophoblast cells were destroyed. (The trypsin specifically broke down the amino acids in the trophoblasts' cell membrane, destroying them.)

Because of this observation, Dr. Beard logically theorized that since "parasitic" trophoblast cells resembled cancer cells in nature, that enzymes would "break down" cancer cells, too.

Dr. Beard set out to prove his theory, and yes, he proved trypsin was effective against cancer cells and tumors.

Dr. Beard first published his findings in 1902 in the distinguished journal, *Lancet*. In the article, Dr. Beard proposed that the enzyme trypsin was the body's main defense against cancer and would be useful as a cancer treatment.

Many scientists and doctors embraced his theory and for the next twenty years, articles were published in medical journals as to the success of enzymes being used to treat cancer.

However, Dr. Beard sadly met strong opposition to his enzyme cancer treatment.

On the positive side, Dr. Beard was nominated for the 1905 Nobel Peace Prize for embryology.

In 1911, Beard published *The Enzyme Treatment of Cancer and Its Scientific Basis*. Released by a major publishing company, the book was soon forgotten by the scientific community, because they had embraced a new cancer "cure"--radiation.

DID YOU KNOW?

Madame Curie died of exposure to her own discovery--uranium.

In 1924, Dr. Beard passed away. Sadly, the allopathic medical community had adopted the slash, poison and burn protocols to treat cancer. It was the beginning of the "Dark Ages" of medicine.

Author's Comments

Dr. Beard was correct in his conclusion that enzymes are one of the body's best defenses against cancer. However, at the time of his research (circa 1890-1902), he probably did not know about mycoplasmas (discovered in 1898) and the "real" reason why enzymes were effective against cancer.

You might have already guessed--why pancreatic enzymes are effective against disease and cancer; but the truth about enzyme therapy is revealed in the next chapter.

The Truth About Enzyme Therapy

The following (partial) editorial appeared in the *New York Times* on October 9, 1909, when newspapers were still "free" presses:

> "In spite of present condemnation of trypsin, there is a large chance that time will tell another story."

It has taken over 100 years for the truth to come out. From Wikipedia:

> "Proponents of Dr. Beard's enzyme theory for the treatment of cancer believe that certain enzymes remove a protective coating from cancer cells, allowing white blood cells to identify and attack them."

The aforementioned is part truth. That protein coating has not replaced the cancer cell's outer surface. The described protein coating is biofilm (plaque) built around the entire mass of cancer cells to protect the colony from the immune system.

When enzymes dissolve the protein plaque, the immune system is then able to break through and destroy the pathogenic colony.

DID YOU KNOW?

Carpal tunnel surgery "scrapes off" the bacterial plaque.

Just like trophoblast cells, bacteria secrete proteases (protein enzymes), referred to as exotoxins, to destroy extracellular structures so they can penetrate and attach to the host's tissues.

Lycozymes

Egg whites contain lycozyme, an enzyme, which protects the chick embryo from bacteria, breaking down bacterial cell walls. It is also found in mother's milk and human tear ducts. Cooking the egg white destroys the enzyme.

Papain

This enzyme is in papaya and used for thousands of years to tenderize meat, mostly in its native habitat, South America. It is also an ingredient in dental products, helping to break down bacterial plaque on teeth.

Bromelain

This enzyme is found in the pineapple, the stem (main stalk), and the leaves of the pineapple plant. The commercial source for the enzyme comes from the stem.

Scientific research has shown that bromelain has the following effects:
- Has anti-tumor and anti-metastisis effects
- Dissolves and reduces formation of blood clots
- Breaks down protein
- Relieves pain
- Reduces inflammation
- Reduces appetite
- Suppresses muscle spasms
- Stuns and/or kills nematodes (roundworms)

The pineapple plant and fruit are plagued by many parasites—viruses, insects, fungi, and bacteria--the whole spectrum.

A phytochemical that acts as a pesticide and affects the central nervous system is an alkaloid or a glucosinolate. Bromelain is not an alkaloid. Scientific studies have not yet identified all alkaloids present in plant(s).

The domesticated pineapple is a descendant of the wild pineapple plant. The wild pineapple plant contains 35,000 parts per million of nitrogen, which re-enforces the presence of alkaloids. A dead give-away that alkaloids are present are studies showing bromelain kills roundworms (a pesticide), relieves pain, suppresses muscle spasms, and reduces inflammation (affects central nervous system).

The supplement bromelain definitely contains "mystery" alkaloid(s) and is an excellent source for killing pathogens and dissolving plaque.

DID YOU KNOW?

Columbus came upon the pineapple in 1493 on the island of Guadeloupe and named it *pina de Indes*, "pine of the Indians." He then brought it back and introduced it to European royalty. Thereafter, royalty in England built greenhouses to grow pineapples. (The pineapple symbolizes wealth.)

Cut off and planted after harvesting, the top of the pineapple grows into a new plant. It takes two years for a plant to mature enough to grow one pineapple.

Forks over Knives

This film is worth watching and is a very good documentary, which re-enforces a plant-based diet reverses disease and cancer.

Researchers in this documentary proved that people who adopt a plant-based diet have less chance of getting cancer and disease compared to people who eat a western diet.

In the documentary, a doctor reversed cardiovascular disease in 18 of his patients by putting them on a plant-based diet. Ten years later, the patients were still on a plant-based diet, healthy and disease-free. Further, two diabetic patients reversed their diabetes by eating a plant-based diet.

The following scientific study, which was quoted in the chapter entitled, "Diseases, Cancers and Conditions Caused by Mycoplasma," would have been proof enough that mycoplasmas are factors or co-factors involved in heart disease:

Arterial Sclerosis: (51)

> 51. Mycoplasmas and Oncogenesis: Persistent Infection and Multistage Malignant Transformation - L. Tsai, et al. Proclamation of National Academy of Sciences, USA, Oct. 24, 1995, 92(22), pp. 10197-10201

Forks over Knives proves the enzyme theory "right on," that not eating meat allows your own pancreatic enzymes to dissolve bacterial plaque and, ultimately, the immune system can reach and kills the pathogens. The body can then heal itself (reverse heart disease).

DID YOU KNOW?

An end product of anaerobic bacterial fermentation is butyrate, which has a very unpleasant odor. Produced by the skin flora (bacteria) under the arms from the fermentation of the lipids in sweat, it is the cause of body odor. Butyrate is what makes feces smell so bad (anaerobic breakdown of fats in the colon). Butyrate (a/k/a/ butyric acid) is in milk.

PDQ Skin Cream

The manufacturers of this topical herbal skin cream are very cautious about making claims that PDQ Skin Cream is effective against skin cancer.

I learned of this product from Lindsey Williams in the documentary *Healing the Elite Way*, where he reveals what the super rich people do to treat cancer.

DID YOU KNOW?

The elite who control this country would NEVER choose radiation or chemo to treat cancer. Instead, they journey down to Mexico to receive treatment.

PDQ skin cream was invented for the elite to treat skin cancer.

The following was taken from Amazon's PDQ product description:

> "We are very careful to not make any claims that the PDQ Herbal Skin Cream will have any effect on dangerous cancer cells, skin cancer, or suspicious skin lesions. We simply rely on hundreds of testimonials from our customers that share with us their amazing results since the products development."

Unfortunately, the ingredients are a trade secret. I am sure, though, that there are alkaloids at work in the cream. Here are the directions from their web site:

> "Results: With only two doses (one drop the first day, another drop 24 hours later), results may be seen as a red bump or a white blister if there is abnormal or dangerous tissue present before the application. Scabbing will occur in another 2 to 3 days and the scab will come off leaving little or no scarring in another 7 to 10 days."

The bottle contains enough to treat ten spots. For more information, visit www.pdqherbals.com.

Heat Therapy

"Give me a fever and I can cure any ailment."

— Hippocrates

Heat therapy is commonly used to treat cancer and disease. Bacteria live comfortably in a temperature ranging from 40° to 140°. They especially like the body temperature of mammals. They prefer a moist and warm environment.

Fever

Fevers are a natural way for the immune system to "cook" pathogens. Experts suggest that patients recover more rapidly from infections or critical illness because of fever.

According to Wikipedia: "Fever assists the healing process in several important ways:

- Increases mobility of leukocytes*
- Enhances phagocytosis*
- Endotoxin effects decreased
- Increased production of T cells"

*See definition at end of chapter.

Author's Comments

Use common sense when monitoring a fever. According to experts, temperatures over 102° for prolonged periods can cause heat seizures.

Biomat

Biomats are FDA approved. They have many health benefits including killing pathogens safely.

Bacteria start dying at 145° and viruses at 160°. The Biomat reaches a maximum temperature of 149°.

The Biomat:

- Alkalizes the body
- Charges the immune system and boosts energy
- Purifies and ionizes the air
- Revitalizes cells
- Helps release stress, tension and anxiety

- Relieves chronic pain and speeds up injury recovery
- Improves circulation and cardiovascular function

Alkalizing the Body

Biomats deliver negative ions directly through the skin's surface via conduction. Calcium and sodium are then ionized. This then changes the blood's pH to alkaline.

Revitalizes the Cells

With negative ions in the blood increasing, inter-cellular communication increases. This results in an increase in cellular nutrient uptake and cellular hydration. This also improves efficiency of the cells being able to dispose of waste.

Reduces Stress and Fatigue

The gentle warmth of the infrared rays helps to sooth nerves and helps relax tight and knotted muscles.

Detoxes

Far infrared helps detox the body of toxins (through sweating) and helps blood circulation.

Kills Bacteria

According to Biomat's specifications, Biomats can reach a temperature of 149°. This is a "safe" zone for humans but a "danger" zone for bacteria.

There are several sizes of Biomats. They come in king size, queen size and single size. There is also a professional size. For more information on Biomats, or to purchase a Biomat, visit the following web site: www.biomatmedical.co

Aromatherapy

Documented aromatherapy has been around for 5,000 years. The Chinese burned herbs to create harmony and well-being. They identified over 300 herbs that have health benefits when burned.

Even the Egyptians used incense, bath oils and massage therapeutically.

Hippocrates, the father of medicine, used aromatic fumigations to rid Athens of the plague. He, too, used aromatherapy and massage in his treatments.

Developed in Arabia, perfume was brought back to Europe by the crusaders.

DID YOU KNOW?

During the Dark Ages, Aromatherapy went underground, because it was thought of as unnatural by the Catholic Church. The church believed illness was punishment from God.

The following are categories in essential oil aromatherapy. They are categorized by scent and their odor:

- <u>Floral:</u> Rose, jasmine, lilac and gardenia
- <u>Citrus:</u> Grapefruit, Mandarin orange, lemon, orange and tangerine
- <u>Mint:</u> Peppermint and spearmint
- <u>Woody:</u> Cedarwood and sandalwood
- <u>Herbaceous:</u> Basil, marjoram and thyme
- <u>Earthy:</u> Oakmoss and patchnoli
- <u>Spicy:</u> Cinnamon, cloves and nutmeg

Lampe Berger

In 1897, a French chemist by the name of Maurice Berger invented a product that improved air quality. Inspired by observing hospitals' stagnant air quality and poor ventilation systems, he was able to receive two patents. One was for the catalytic burner and the other for Ozoalcool, which is still to this day a trade secret.

Ozoalcool

Maurice Berger used Isopropyl Alcohol in his aromatherapy invention extracted from French beetroot and refined into white sugar and then into Isopropyl alcohol. This type of water-soluble alcohol blends easily with essential oils.

Wikipedia, describes Ozoalcool and how the lamp works as follows:

> "When dissolved in liquid form, the ozoalcool and isopropyl alcohol blend together. As a gas, oxygen anion (O) will be added into the molecular structure of the Isopropyl alcohol to form isopropyl ozoacool. Ozoalcool will release oxygen under the process of catalyzed oxidation and will combine with oxygen molecules in the atmosphere to become supercharged oxygen. This supercharged oxygen is commonly known as ozone. As a powerful oxidizing agent, it will eliminate unpleasant odors and secondhand smoke, acting also as an anti-microbial agent. Through the natural oxidation process in which the extra oxygen anion in the ozone combines with the atoms of the offending odor/toxin oxidizing it and leaving only oxygen in its place. Thus, the air is left fresh and clean smelling."

DID YOU KNOW?

The following are some fun facts about our sense of smell:

- Studies show that 75% of emotions are triggered by smell.
- The sense of smell is fully developed in the womb.
- A woman's sense of smell is stronger than a man's sense of smell.
- We can smell things better in the spring and summer because of moisture in the air.
- Humans have five to six million smell-detecting cells. Rabbits have 100 million and dogs have a whopping 220 million.
- The smell of a new car is one of the most popular scents.

Purchasing a Lamp Berger is worth investigating. They are available on the Internet.

Phage Therapy

Once the medical industry recognizes that cancer and disease are most commonly bacterial infections, this type of therapy would be an effective inexpensive treatment.

The Discovery of Bacteriophages

As far back as records go, there were reports that river water had the ability to "cure" infectious diseases such as leprosy.

In 1896, Ernest Hambury Hankin observed a phenomenon. He reported something in the waters of India's rivers had antibacterial actions against cholera.

Then in 1915, Frederick Twort, a bacteriologist, discovered an agent that killed bacteria. He theorized it was either an enzyme or a virus or just a stage in the life cycle of the bacteria. Unfortunately, WWI interrupted his research.

In 1917, Felix d'Herelle of the Louis Pasteur Institute discovered an invisible and antagonistic microbe--a virus parasite on bacteria. He called this virus a bacteriophage (from Greek *phage* meaning to eat). He documented a patient being cured of dysentery using bacteriophages. Felix is now known as the researcher who introduced the concept of phage therapy.

Bacteriophages were discovered to be anti-bacterial and used in the United States and in Georgia (Russia) in the 1920s and 1930s. However, with the introduction of antibiotics in the 1950s, the American medical industry lost interest in phage therapy. (Drugs were more profitable and the #1 choice for the treatment of disease and cancer.)

According to sources, there are nineteen families of viruses, which attack bacteria.

Unfortunately, antibiotics kill <u>both</u> good and bad bacteria; but bacteriophages are very specific, targeting only certain strains of bacteria.

DID YOU KNOW?

Bacteriophages have killed antibiotic-resistant bacteria that cause pneumonia.

One of the densest places to find phages is in the ocean. Scientists estimate that 70 percent of bacteria living in the oceans are infected with bacteriophages.

For the last 90 years, phage therapy has been used as an alternative to antibiotics in Georgia (part of the former Soviet Union), in central Europe, and in France.

Communist Russia in the early 20th century has a most interesting tale to tell regarding phage research.

George Eliava Institute of Bacteriophage

Professor George Eliava was unaware of bacteriophages until he visited the Louis Pasteur Institute in Paris and met Felix d'Herelle. Eliava was so fascinated with the concept of phage therapy that he invited d'Herelle to Georgia to visit his bacteriology laboratory.

Felix d'Herelle visited the laboratory twice in 1933-1934. In 1934, Stalin invited d'Herelle to work at the bacteriological institute and d'Herelle accepted. He worked with the Russians for 18 months.

In 1935, d'Herelle dedicated one of his books on phage therapy to Stalin. In 1937, d'Herelle was planning on taking up permanent residence on the grounds of the institute; but before he moved to Georgia, tragedy struck.

George Eliava, accused of being an enemy of the people, was put to death by Stalin. This squashed d'Herelle's plans to work at the institute. (Even though Eliava was dead, the institute of phage therapy stayed open.)

During the days of the "Iron Curtain," people from all over Russia came to the institute for treatment of cancer and disease. Phage therapy had become routine practice throughout Russia for the treatment of bacterial infections.

In 1991, Georgia refused to become part of the Russian Federation and war broke out in Georgia. The institute was destroyed, along with its records and bacteriophage samples.

Then in 1997, a report was broadcast on the English BBC, which sparked an interest in phage therapy. The institute took several years to recover, thanks to scientists and doctors who flocked to Georgia to aid in salvaging this type of therapy. Visit their web site:

www.eliava-institute.org

DID YOU KNOW

In August 2001, an article appeared in the *Journal of Microbiology* entitled "Transduction by φBB-1, a Bacteriophage of Borrelia burgdorferi," co-authored by the US government.

I ask, "Why has a taxpayer-funded government agency (NIH) kept an effective treatment for Lyme disease buried for over 15 years, when millions of people worldwide are suffering (and dying) from Lyme disease?"

Summary

The following are my "picks" for the most effective treatments against bacteria, fungus, and viruses:

Bacteria and Fungus

*Mild silver protein IV (20,000 ppm)

Mild silver protein drops by mouth or nebulizer (20,000 ppm)

Goldenseal

Bloodroot, Vinca Minor, Oleander, Nicotine Patch

Rife Machine and Zapper

Ozone and Vitamin C IV therapy

Viruses

Goldenseal

AUTHOR'S FINAL COMMENT

A ketogenic diet is of <u>absolute</u> necessity when fighting an infection, especially mycoplasma, Candida and Lyme disease.

All of these protocols in this book are not a "cure." A person can get re-infected with mycoplasma, the Lyme spirochaete and other pathogens, including viruses.

*Mild silver protein is ineffective against eliminating tumors. Mild silver protein is a "natural" one-time antibiotic that does not kill the good bacteria in your gut.

Sources

Both www.wikipedia.org and Dr. Duke's Phytochemical and Ethnobotanical Databases were the major source for <u>all</u> categories. Articles are in quotes. Movies, magazines and books are italicized. (Sources are not mentioned twice, if referenced in chapter.)

MYCOPLASMA

US Patent, *AIDS Made in America"* Common Cause Medical Research Foundation Journal, Donald W. Scott

"MYCOPLASMA: The Linking Pathogen in Neurosystemic Diseases" Donald W. Scott, *Nexus Magazine* Aug 2001

Amyotrophic Lateral Sclerosis by Donald W. Scott and William L.C. Scott

The Brucellosis Triangle by Donald W. Scott and William L.C. Scott

The Journal of Degenerative Diseases, Volume 7, Number 2, Fall 2006, AIDS, Part 2 and Watergate – Common Cause Research Foundation

The Journal of Degenerative Diseases, Volume 4, Number 4, Autumn 2003, The Sudbury Study – Common Cause Research Foundation

The Journal of Degenerative Diseases, Volume 5, Number 3, Summer 2003, AIDS, Made in America– Common Cause Research Foundation

The Journal of Degenerative Diseases, Volume 6, Number 1&2, Spring/Summer 2005/ Sxth Annual Conference Edition– Common Cause Research Foundation

The Journal of Degenerative Diseases, Volume 3, Number 1, July 2001 "X" Marks the Spot– Common Cause Research Foundation

The Journal of Degenerative Diseases, Volume 4, Number 1, July 2002– Common Cause Research Foundation

The Journal of Degenerative Diseases, Volume 7, Number 3, Spring 2007, AIDS and the Deep Politics of the United States – Common Cause Medical Research Foundation

MYCOPLASMA PHOTOS

Dr. Harold Clark (deceased), Mycoplasma Research Institute, Beverly Hills, FL

CANCER AND DISEASE

"What Causes Cancer" by R. Webster Kehr, Independent Cancer Research Foundation, Inc., www.cancertutor.com

CANCER, DISEASES & CONDITIONS/MYCOPLASMA

The Journal of Degenerative Diseases, Vol 5, No. 1, Winter 2003 edition by the Common Cause Medical Research Foundation

SPIROCHAETES

Journal of Bacteriology, August 2001

PLANT PHYTOCHEMICAL MOLECULAR STRUCTURE

www.chemicalbook.com and www.pubchem.gov

BOVINE COLOSTRUM

"Colostrum is a Proven, Effective Immune System Booster" by Danny Veracity

THE STORY OF DR. HAZEL PARCELLS

www.parcellscenter.com

"Parcells Oxygen Soak and Water Purification" by Joseoh Dispenza

TOBACCO

"Nicotine Patches in Alzheimer's Disease Pilot Study on Learning, Memory and Safety," AL Wilson, LK Langley, T Bauer, S Rottunda, E McFalls, C Kovera, JR McCarten, Dept. of Veteran's Affairs Medical Center, Minneapolis, MN

"Nicotine Treatment of Mild Cognitive Impairment - A 6-month double-blind pilot clinical trial," Georgetown University, Vanderbilt, University of California-San Diego, and Duke--P Newhouse, K Kellar, P Aisen, H White

MARIJUANA

"Hemp Oil: Another Suppressed Cancer Cure" by Rick Simpson

The Marijuana Movie

Run from the Cure, a movie documentary about Rick Simpson

"Hemp Protein: Eat the Nutrients" by Amiellia Ponds, www.naturalnews.com

"Anhydrocannabisativine, a New Alkaloid from Cannabis sativa, MA Elsohly, CE Turner, CH Phoebe, JE Knapp, PL Schiff, Jr., DJ Slatkin

"Isolation of Cannabisativine, an Alkaloid from Cannabis sativa root," CE Turner, MH Hsu, JE Knapp, PL Schiff, Jr., DJ Slatkin

THE STORY OF HEMP-EAZE

Darcy Stoddard's blog, www.hemp-eaze.com

HEMP SEEDS

"Hemp and Haw No More" by Peter Benner, Summer 2000 issue of *The Gilded Herb magazine*, Volume 2, Issue 2

"Hemp Seed: The Most Nutritionally Complete Food Source in the World, Part One and Part Two" by Lynn Osburn

CINNAMON

"Eleven Health Benefits of Cinnamon" by Andrea Manitsas

"Popular Chewing Gum Eliminates Bacteria That Cause Bad Breath," *ScienceDaily*, April 2004

OLEANDER

"Oleander" by R. Webster Kehr, Independent Cancer Research Foundation, Inc., www.cancertutor.com

Cancer's Natural Enemy (ebook) by Tony Isaacs

"A Natural Anti-Cancer Protocol" by Tony Isaacs

"The Mysteries of the Cancer Fighting Oleander Plant" by Tony Isaacs

TURMERIC AND GINGER

"Alzheimer's Disease - Natural Treatment with Spices" by Keith Scott, M.D.

ESSIAC TEA

"The Story of Essiac Tea," www.bulk-essiac-tea.com

HOXSEY THERAPY

"The Hoxsey Therapy or Hoxsey Method," www.cureyourself.co.uk

"Alternative Cancer Therapies," Wellness Directory of Minnesota[TM] www.mnwelldir.org

AMYGDALIN/LAETRILE

"Naturally Occurring Toxicants as Etiologic Agents of Foodborne Disease" by Gregory Moller, Ph.D.

"Laetrile and the Life Saving Substance Called Cyanide" by Philp Binzel, Jr., M.D.

"Fruit and Vegetables that Produce Cyanide," www.inspection.gc.ca

"Foods Containing B17 (Nitrilosides)," www.vitaminb17.org

World Without Cancer, a documentary by G. Edward Griffith

"The Nitrilosides in Plants and Animals - Nutritional & Therapeutic Implications" by Ernst T. Krebs, John Beard Memorial Foundation

MORINGA

"Contribution to the Study of the Anti-Inflammatory Activity of Moringa oleifera," M Ndiaye, AM Dieye, F Mariko, AQ Tall, A Sall Diallo, B Faye, 2002

"An Anti-Tumor Promoter from Moringa oleifera," AP Guevara, C Vargas, H Sakurai, Y Fujiwara, K Hashimoto, T Maoka, M Kozuika, Y Ito, H Tokuda, H Nishino

"Moringa oleifera: A Review of the Medicinal Evidence for its Nutritional, Therapeutic and Prophylactic Properties," JW Fahey

"Moringa oleifera: A Food with Multiple Medicinal Uses," F Anwar, S Latif, F Ashraf, AH Gilani, 2007

MEDIUM-CHAIN FATTY ACIDS

Coconut Cures by Bruce Fife, N.D.

The Coconut Oil Miracle by Bruce Fifte, N.D.

"Coconut Oil in Health and Disease: Its Monolaurin's Potential as Cure for HIV/AIDS" by Conrado S. Dayrit, M.D.

"Cocos Nucifera," by Karen Smith

"Coconut Oil-Arthritis" by Bruce Fife, N.D.

"There is a Cure for Arthritis" by Bruce Fife, N.D.

"The Fat That Can Make You Thin" by Bruce Fife, N.D.

"Coconut Water: Dew from the Heavens" by Bruce Fife, N.D.

GERSON THERAPY

The Gerson Miracle Movie

ENERGY THERAPY

"Royal Rife: Cancer Cure Genius Silenced by Medical Mafia" by Paul Fassa

"The Cancer Cure that Worked, Fifty Years of Suppression" by Deki and John C. Fox, www.educate-yourself.org

The Cancer Cure that Worked by Barry Lynes

"Treating Cancer" by Ken Adachi, www.educate-yourself.org

"Using Zapper to Kill Parasites that May Lie Behind Cancers" by Ginny Fraser

BAKING SODA

"My Dance with Cancer" by Vernon "Vito" Johnson, www.phkillscancer.com

"Living Proof - an Alternative Prostate Cancer Treatment," www.canceractive.com

SILVER

"The Truth About Covalent Silver," www.silver-colloids.com

"Bacteriology Studies of Ionic Silver are Bogus," www.silver-colloids.com

"How to Tell if a Product is Mostly Ionic Silver," www.silver-colloids.com

"How to Compare Colloidal Silver Products," www.silver-colloids.com

"The Truth About Ionic Silver," www.silver-colloids.com

"A Layman's Guide to Using Colloidal Silver" by Ben Taylor

SULFUR

"The Importance of the MSM Protocols" by R. Webster Kehr, Independent Cancer Research Foundation, Inc., www.cancertutor.com

"Fact: Bad Bacteria Cannot Survive in an Oxygen-Rich Environment" - www.h2oairwateramericas.com

"Organic Sulfur - The Deliverance Mineral for All Manner of Sickness (MSM)" by Gregory Ciola, www.utopiasilver.com

HEAT THERAPY

www.biomatmedical.com

VENUS FLYTRAP

"What is Carnivora? - www.carnivora.com

Definition of Wisdom

Knowledge is not intelligence and intelligence is not wisdom. Knowledge is nothing more than an amassed familiarity with facts. These facts can be of any number of things, i.e., scientific findings, mathematical principles, history, politics, etc. All it tells us is that a person has the ability to remember a great deal of information/facts.

The next aspect of this equation is intelligence or the ability to understand facts and their inter-dependent relationship to each other.

Just knowing facts does not allow someone to make the connection between them. That takes intelligence and unfortunately this is where the majority of people stop. They believe that intelligence is the end of knowing. It isn't.

Knowledge requires wisdom for it to be harmonious and beneficial. The problem with wisdom is that it cannot be learned through science, reason or logic.

True wisdom can only be gained through experience and when all desires to achieve personal profit, presence and power have been eliminated. It can also be gained through self-sacrifice and suffering.

– Unknown Source

Made in the USA
San Bernardino, CA
11 January 2017